INTERMITTENT FASTING SUCCESS STORY

HOW I LOST 110 POUNDS AND WILL NEVER DIET AGAIN!

Paige Davidson

©Copyright 2022 by Action Takers Publishing™

All rights reserved. No part of this book may be reproduced or transmitted in any form or by any electronic or mechanical means, including photocopying, recording or by any information storage and retrieval system, without the written permission of the publisher, except where permitted by law.

Action Takers Publishing™
www.actiontakerspublishing.com

Paperback ISBN: 978-1-7348759-8-0
eBook ISBN: 978-1-7348759-9-7

NOTE: The information in this book is not intended or implied to be a substitute for professional medical advice, diagnosis, or treatment. Always consult your physician before beginning any exercise or diet program. This work is not intended to diagnose any medical condition or to replace your healthcare professional. Consult with your healthcare professional to design an appropriate diet and exercise prescription.

Cover Design by Sam Art Studio
Printed in the United States of America

TABLE OF CONTENTS

Foreword by Dr. Mark Mattson v
Introduction 1

PART I | INTERMITTENT FASTING IS DIET FREEDOM: FACT OR FICTION?
Chapter 1 | Breaking the Grip of the Diet Curse 11
Chapter 2 | Intermittent Fasting 101 17
Chapter 3 | Reset Your Health for Life 27

PART II | ONE PAIGE AT A TIME
Chapter 4 | Goal Setting Sets You Free.. 35
Chapter 5 | Measures of Success 43
Chapter 6 | Breaking Free of Food Addiction 49

PART III | THE NEXT PAIGE
Chapter 7 | The Power of Habits 57
Chapter 8 | Good Habits Changed My Story 65
Chapter 9 | Bad Behaviors Breakdown 73

PART IV | PAIGE TURNER
Chapter 10 | Self-Love & Self-Care... 83
Chapter 11 | Mindset Matters! 91
Chapter 12 | Movement: the Other Fountain............................... 101
of Youth
Epilogue 109

FOREWORD
DR. MARK MATTSON

The epidemics of childhood and adult obesity have occurred as a result of the consumption of excessive amounts of calories and lack of exercise. People with obesity want to lose weight and most attempt to do so by trying calorie-counting diet plans. But this may actually cause them to obsess about everything they eat all day every day. And once a person has developed obesity, their brain has changed in ways that exacerbate the problem. Their brain no longer responds well to leptin – the satiety hormone. As a result, they perceive that they are hungry when a normal weight person would feel full. Moreover, people can actually become addicted to food as has been shown by scientists who study what happens in the addicted brain. Particularly addictive are the kinds of highly palatable foods loaded with sugars and fats that are readily available and intensively marketed by the companies that produce them.

I expect most people never asked themselves why they eat breakfast, lunch, dinner, and a snack every day. The answer turns out to be simple – that's what their parents and folks in their workplace do. It is with this traditional eating pattern that people have become obese. Why? Because with this eating pattern a person may never tap their fat stores and so the fat continues to accumulate. In contrast, when a person ceases eating for 16 hours or more, they switch to a fat burning mode. Doing this every day will enable them to lose weight. Controlled trials have shown that this and other intermittent fasting eating patterns are effective for weight loss in people with obesity.

In this book, Paige Davidson tells her remarkable and compelling personal story of her struggle with morbid obesity during which she embarked on many different calorie-counting diets without success. She was finally able to get her weight into the normal range by switching to an intermittent fasting eating pattern in which she consumed all of her food within a 6-hour time window every day. I am a neuroscientist and so was particularly fascinated by Paige's detailed descriptions of the psychological impact of her obesity and why calorie-counting diets only made things worse. With an engaging writing style, she recounts her emotional struggles, how they affected her relationships, and how intermittent fasting enabled her to overcome these problems. She provides valuable tips for fine-tuning a lifestyle that includes intermittent fasting. This is a must read for anyone with obesity. It will provide them with motivation, encouragement, and a clear path to the light at the end of the tunnel.

Longstanding obesity is a major contributor to early deaths from heart disease, stroke, diabetes, and many cancers. It also increases one's risk for depression, cognitive impairment, and Alzheimer's disease. During the past 35 years, my research at the University of Kentucky, the National Institute on Aging, and Johns Hopkins University has been aimed at understanding what goes wrong in the brain in Alzheimer's and Parkinson's diseases and if and how one might reduce their risk for these devastating diseases. We discovered that intermittent fasting was very effective in protecting brain cells and preventing neurological deficits in animal models of Alzheimer's and Parkinson's diseases. Moreover, we showed that intermittent fasting can improve glucose regulation, reduce blood pressure, lower inflammation, improve mood, and enhance learning and memory. As detailed in my recent book, *The Intermittent Fasting Revolution*, we have learned much about how intermittent fasting bolsters the resilience of cells in the body and brain. As I read Paige Davidson's fascinating personal story,

I imagined these same changes occurring in the cells of her body and brain. It is gratifying to learn about people such as her for whom intermittent fasting has proven to be a life saver.

Mark P. Mattson, Ph.D.
Adjunct Professor of Neuroscience, Johns Hopkins University School of Medicine
Former Chief of the Laboratory of Neurosciences at the National Institute on Aging

INTRODUCTION

As I was waiting in the drive through of a popular fast-food restaurant, a car full of adolescent boys drove slowly past me, hurling trash at my car and screaming obscenities and phrases that included "fat pig" and "Yeah, eat more and get even fatter, you hog!" Humiliation and embarrassment kept me from picking up my lunch order. I couldn't face the look of pity on the poor restaurant employee's face as I sped past the window. I couldn't escape fast enough, trying to hide the tears that amplified my shame.

Abject cruelty. The only experience that is worse than the invisibility morbidly obese women suffer in today's society. After this cruel incident, I almost welcomed the familiar invisibility that I wore like a cloak daily. Morbid obesity in America is considered a character flaw. It feels humiliating to know that you are assumed to be stupid, at best, because how else could you allow yourself to become so fat. Pretending not to see the look of disgust on interviewers' faces, knowing that you will be passed over for yet another job that you are highly qualified for, is degrading and beyond disheartening. To know that the reason you are invisible to others is because they have no respect for you, they see you as less than, they assume that you are dirty, or slovenly, and even lazy, is to feel constant dejection and hopelessness.

I grew up in diet culture, both in my home and in society. I learned early on that in order to lose weight, you had to "go somewhere." Some diet doctor had to fix you, to tell you what to do, what to eat and not to eat. For over 40 years, I tried every weight loss center in existence. I began my weight loss attempts in high school, falling into a vicious cycle that would continue for many years with this same weekly weigh-in program. I joined, hopeful this would be the time that it would work.

INTRODUCTION

I tried my best for a while, suffering the embarrassment and growing sense of failure each week as I was weighed, expected to report my progress (or lack thereof) that week to the rest of the group, and I would eventually quit. Until the next time I was called fat, or ignored in a situation that particularly stung, or got so winded trying to climb a set of stairs that it frightened me. Then the cycle would begin again, the same process playing itself out as my self-esteem plummeted, until it was eventually non-existent.

Decades worth of various diets, exercise programs, doctor supervised liquid diets, physician prescribed weight loss pills, injections of who knows what, potions hyped to be "the solution," and diets that eliminated entire food groups later, weighing over 300 pounds and physically and emotionally broken, I desperately submitted to my most extreme weight-loss attempt: gastric bypass surgery. At age 37, this was one of the scariest things I had ever considered doing, but I felt it was necessary if I wanted any semblance of a life. I was the 2nd gastric bypass surgery patient in Kentucky in 2000. I will never forget the surgeon saying to me, "Paige, I can operate on your stomach, but I can't operate on your brain." And that was it! There was no further information or assistance given in this area.

Hearing this was terrifying because I knew exactly what he meant, and yet I knew nothing at all about what he meant. Clearly there was something wrong with my thinking, but what? When you have thought the same way since you were a child, you believe that it's just the way it is; what everyone thinks. What is normal. I absolutely could not identify how my thinking was flawed, or caused me to gain then lose, then gain then lose, ad nauseum. The first step in healing is always awareness. How can you heal from disordered thinking when you have no idea how your thinking is disordered?

Providing me with the physical tool to assist me with weight loss yet failing to provide me with the tools to change the lifestyle, mindset, attitude, and disordered thinking that led to morbid obesity in the first place was irresponsible healthcare. Yet who did I blame when the surgery was ultimately a failure? Myself, of course! Never mind the fact that if I had known how to cure myself all on my own, I would never have been morbidly obese in the first place. Meanwhile, my sense of failure continued to snowball.

Knowing that I was dying a slow death, one forkful at a time, I desperately set out to do something I had never done before; try to get healthy, not just lose weight. The very first thing I did was to declare that I was never going to diet again! Forty years of dieting had resulted in me weighing 315 pounds at the time of my ill-fated weight loss surgery. You could say I "dieted" my way up to 315 pounds. I wasn't sure exactly how to proceed, but I did know for sure that a diet was not the answer.

I also decided to try another thing I had never tried before, counseling. I was 56 years old and still riding the weight loss/gain rollercoaster. I found a good fit with an amazing Christian counselor named Linda, and at our first meeting, I told her "There is something really wrong with me. I either have a food addiction, or an eating disorder, or maybe I have OCD when it comes to food and eating. But regardless of what it is, I have to get it figured out, because I just can't continue to live my life this way!"

Soon after Linda and I began our work, I learned of intermittent fasting (IF), which is an amazingly healthy way of eating and managing food. IF is not a diet, although I did not believe that at first. In fact, I declared that it sounded like yet another crazy fad diet, and I wasn't doing it! However, I soon learned that besides not being a fad OR a diet, it actually heals inflammation in your body. This got my attention, because I was suffering with acute pain due to plantar fasciitis in one foot, and Achilles' Tendonitis in the other. I was in such severe, constant pain that I was limping. It was debilitating. Inflammation drives both conditions, and this particular side effect of practicing an

INTRODUCTION

IF lifestyle captured my attention. After researching IF, I discovered that it isn't indicated for those who have a history of eating disorders. Concerned, I brought my research to Linda and expressed my interest in trying IF. Not to lose weight, although by then I was back up to 250 pounds, 19 years after my bypass surgery, precipitating my desire to begin counseling. Linda reminded me that we had no idea yet if I had an eating disorder or not and suggested that I try fasting, and if I found it helpful, continue it. If I don't, just stop doing it.

With her blessing, I began right away. Briefly for now, to practice an IF lifestyle is merely to eat your food within a period of time each day, called an eating window. Outside of your eating window you practice a clean fast. For example, one popular IF protocol is 18/6. Fast for 18 hours (including sleeping time) and consume your food during your six-hour eating window. IF attends to when you eat your food, not what you eat. You focus on eating foods that you enjoy and that are good for you, and throw in an occasional treat, whatever that means to you.

Within two weeks, my pain was reduced enough that I was no longer limping. I could walk normally! Within six months, my painful foot conditions were 100% healed. And even more incredibly, I had also lost almost 55 pounds! Finally accepting that intermittent fasting really was not a diet, I came to the shocking conclusion that I actually could lose weight without going somewhere, looking for someone to fix me. After 40 years of yo-yo dieting, I was finally succeeding at becoming healthy while losing weight at the same time. Life is good.

Practicing an IF lifestyle was the beginning of an amazing new sense of empowerment, to take my health and wellness into my own hands. I kept going, and in 14 months had lost 110 pounds and many clothing sizes. Yet this weight loss was a mere footnote to this story compared to the other benefits practicing IF brought me.

I learned to be an intuitive eater, learning to focus on healthy foods that I loved, that made me feel amazing. I learned the importance of a positive attitude and mindset. I discovered that healthy habits are foundational to a healthy lifestyle, and I learned the critical lesson of what it means to truly love myself! Of deep importance was the fact that I actually learned how to stop the negative, mean self-talk, and learned to show myself lots of grace, to be kind and loving and gentle with myself. This made all the difference in the world in the way I felt about myself and even my outlook on life! You will learn more details about these as you read further. What I thought was yet another weight loss journey turned out to be a deeply spiritual journey with physical healing. Ultimately, I learned that by becoming empowered to make good decisions for myself, I truly went from being invisible in the world, to being invincible – as a woman who was fully in charge of her own physical, mental, emotional, and spiritual health!

Over the past few years, I discovered that shifts in mindset and lifestyle have everything to do with losing weight and keeping it off. I learned that we have the power over our mindset and there are two kinds of lifestyles: the kind you choose, and the kind that you allow to choose you. I hope this book helps you become empowered to change your mindset and choose what kind of lifestyle you are going to live, and that it guides you toward doing so.

As of this writing, I am 59 years old. I started IF at the age of 56 and still experience wonderful benefits of practicing intermittent fasting every day. Food no longer has the hold on me that it once did. I decided to dedicate my life to helping others learn the same lessons that I learned along the way as I lost 110 pounds. Toward that end, I became a certified health and life coach, specializing in intermittent fasting and mindset work. I started a virtual business providing coaching services to those around the world who want to finally lose weight and become healthy and happy. You will find that this book closely follows along with my 12-week coaching program, which can be found at www.FastingWithPaige.com.

As you read, you will also learn that I am very transparent and share many lessons I learned along the way, mistakes I made so you can avoid those sand traps, and an additional lesson I learned after I reached my goal. We are all real people, with real lives, stresses, pressures, and struggles. Relapses can, in fact, happen. What do you do when you come face-to-face with this reality? More on that in the epilogue of this book, along with the fact that the comeback is always greater than the setback!

When you picked up this book, the first question you had was undoubtedly, "What kind of diet do I have to do?" Here is the surprising answer: NONE! You are not going to diet. In fact, you are never going to do another diet, ever! The reason is simple: diets DO NOT work!

Because it is not just about losing weight. It is about losing the mindset and lifestyle that got you there in the first place. And it is about making shifts and adjustments in your fasting lifestyle as you live your life.

You absolutely CAN do this; let's do it together!

A SNAPSHOT OF MY WEIGHT GAIN AND FLUCTUATION	**WEIGHT**
1978 (15 years old) Started first commercial diet program	135
1981 (18 years old) Still quitting/ rejoining the same diet program	165
1984 (21 years old) Got married, tried another diet program	155

1988 (25 years old) Had first baby, joined a gym and another diet program	205 (gained 50 pounds)
1994 (31 years old) Had second baby, went back to the weekly weigh-in diet program in which I participated in 1978	262 (gained 25 pounds)
1997 (34 years old) Got divorced, have now tried 4 more diet programs, with weight fluctuating wildly	293
2000 (37 years old) Had weight loss surgery, weighing the most I'd ever weighed	315
2003 (40 years old) Lost 150 pounds	165
2010 (47 years old) Kept weight off about 4 1/2 years, regaining weight and panicking – tried another diet program	218
2017 (54 years old) Continuing to gain and panic, went back to the 1978 diet program –again.	235
2019 (56 years old) Discovered and began practicing IF	249
2020 (57 years old) Lost 110 pounds. My weight was actually too low, so I worked on correcting that	139
2022 (59 years old) Had a very stressful COVID experience, regained more than intended, but IF always has my back, and all is well	179

Okay. Let's get started!

PART I

INTERMITTENT FASTING IS DIET FREEDOM: FACT OR FICTION?

Chapter 1

BREAKING THE GRIP OF THE DIET CURSE

The curse, as I thought of it, began in childhood. For many years, as far back as elementary school, I felt that I had to be on a diet. I didn't think there was even a choice. To me, this was just a fact. As I got older, the feeling I had was that of being chained to dieting. I certainly felt shackled, that I had no choice in or freedom from this pursuit of the perfect diet. I didn't like dieting and was much happier when I was not on a diet, free to eat all the yummy stuff that I really wanted, but it never occurred to me that it didn't have to be this way. This was clearly a belief that I held, despite the fact that I was convinced it was a truth, not a belief. Ultimately, this core belief led me to diet my way up to 315 pounds.

Around my house, dieting was ever present, as far back as I can remember. Looking back, I understand that it was the culture in my family. It seemed to consume daily life and affected so many things. What we ate, how we grocery shopped, and what kinds of foods we purchased, what kinds of snacks we were allowed to have, going with my mother to her weekly weigh-in dieting program, and on and on. How we ate often depended on how Mom was doing on her diet. If it was a good week there were no trips to the ice cream shop, or snack cakes purchased at the grocery store, or soft drinks allowed. But if Mom was having a hard time and not sticking to her diet, then I really had a good time with those kinds of treats that weren't always allowed in our house. I was overjoyed when Mom had a snack of ice cream or chips, because that meant that I was allowed to follow suit. If we went to visit family, and they offered us a piece of homemade cake, I waited anxiously to see if Mom accepted a piece, hoping she would so I could have some, too. If she didn't accept a piece, I didn't dare accept one. Looking back, I don't ever remember her telling me I couldn't have the cake; I just knew not to, if she didn't have any. These were self-imposed thoughts and restrictions, but I didn't realize it at the time.

As I got older, I realized that my two sisters didn't seem to have the same feelings about food that I did. They ate however they wanted, no matter what Mom was eating. This was a shocking revelation to me. While my food choices and eating patterns were strongly tied to whatever Mom was doing, my sisters didn't seem to care, or to even pay attention to what Mom was eating, or not eating. It was clear that I loved food, and Mom saw this early on. Mom's side of the family dealt with obesity and morbid obesity. Not every single family member, but most of Mom's family struggled with weight just like Mom did. Dad was downright skinny, and his whole family was as well. Mom was an amazing woman. Smart, determined, hard-working, and observant. One thing she observed was that while I loved food and eating, neither of my sisters cared that much about what they ate. Mom had traveled a hard road in her lifelong struggle with obesity. While I was a normal weight as a child, Mom wasn't, and had been overweight even as a young child. Mom became very concerned for me, because she feared that I was heading down that same dark path of struggle with food and weight that she had, and she desperately wanted to save me from that fate.

This was why my eating was so tied to what Mom was doing. Not only was I observing everything she was doing, but she also began to watch everything I ate and began to make comments about what things I should and shouldn't eat. She noticed if I wanted to eat foods that were not on her diet, and she deemed them to be bad foods that would make me fat if I didn't quit eating them. Unfortunately, I was a stubborn child and chafed against these food rules. My solution was to sneak foods that I wanted. You don't want me to eat these crackers? Then I'll sneak them into my room and hide them and eat them when I want! Of course, I always got caught doing this, which made things much worse and set us up to argue about food.

When I was either in middle school or high school, at Mom's urging, I joined the same weekly weight-loss program she followed. I would lose, then cheat on the diet, then gain, and so forth, the beginnings of a lifetime of yo-yo dieting.

By the time I was in college, Mom had lost over 100 pounds on that weekly weigh-in program. She was within a few pounds of her goal when she quit going, and subsequently regained the 100+ pounds. I had done the same thing with about 25 pounds. At that point, she began attending other diet programs, doing other diets like the cabbage soup diet, and the hot dog and ice cream diet, Atkins, South-beach, physician weight loss programs, etc. Ultimately, she lost and then regained 100 pounds three different times, on three different diets. I always followed her to each diet program, each diet center, each gym, until I tried even more things than she did, like physician prescribed weight loss medications, injections of who knows what at one diet facility, and weight-loss surgery. The owner of one weight-loss center called me a "professional dieter" when he took my dieting history and heard all the different interventions I had tried. Each time losing some weight, hanging on until I couldn't hang on or live with the restrictions anymore, then gaining the weight back plus more.

Do I blame my mom for any of this? Absolutely not! I was raised by a strong mother who never gave up and kept trying to lose the excess weight and be healthy. She was one of a generation of women who watched the actions of their own mother and learned these same behaviors. Mom was genuinely doing the very best she could to help me avoid a lifetime of misery with weight and food issues. She, like thousands of other mothers at the time, didn't realize that mothers are their children's first and best teacher when it comes to food and eating issues, and that children learn so many habits and patterns just from observation, as well as direct instruction. We all do the best we can, and there is no doubt that Mom was doing her best to help me. I love her for her dedication to trying to make my life better than hers had been!

When I began my intermittent fasting journey at 56, the first thing I had to do was establish my "why." At first, that was an easy call. Pure and simple, I was in pain. My only reason to start practicing intermittent fasting was because of the inflammation-driven foot conditions that were causing me so much pain. My why was to be able to walk without limping. Since I achieved that goal within two weeks, I doubled down on my why and vowed to heal these foot conditions and become completely pain-free. Weight and losing weight were not connected to my why at all at that point. Within 6 months, I had not only cured the painful foot conditions, but I had cured Obstructive Sleep Apnea, greatly improved my skin, my energy was through the roof, the dreaded brain fog disappeared, AND I had lost almost 55 pounds! Finally understanding that intermittent fasting was not a diet, but a true lifestyle, it was time to amend my why and make it more relevant to my life and my situation. It was only after I understood that I wasn't dieting but living a healthy lifestyle that I could begin to search my feelings and thoughts to find out why I wanted to lose weight. Sure, there were lots of superficial reasons. I wanted all the clothes in my closet to fit. Shoot, I wanted those clothes to be much smaller sizes. I wanted to look good, even though I had quit worrying about trying to be skinny years ago. When my youngest son graduated from college, I wanted to be able to find an amazing outfit to wear to the graduation ceremony. More soul searching revealed that these were great goals to try to meet along the way, but none of them were my true why. Down deep, what was my true north, my real reason to want to release this weight, once and for all?

I intuitively knew that it had to be more meaningful to my life than these goals that I had identified. I finally came to realize that what was at stake if I did not release this weight was my physical, emotional, and mental health and well-being. I longed to live a long, healthy life, free of the aches and pains that I had been suffering from for years and be fully present for the milestones in my children's lives, like career achievements, marriage, and parenthood. I wanted to live my own life fully, and as they say, "die young…as late as possible."

These thoughts and feelings were deep, and I realized that I had identified my why. To gain holistic health, vitality and longevity were the reasons that I wanted to lose this weight. Your why must be deeply meaningful for you. A desire that won't go away once you meet smaller goals such as changing clothing sizes or buying a special outfit for a special event. Your why has to sustain you for life, well past the point of reaching a weight loss goal. It must be your life goal.

Now that I have your attention regarding intermittent fasting, think long and hard about your why. What is that deep-seated need that finally losing the weight, once and for all, will fulfill? I have stated that intermittent fasting is not a diet. So, what exactly is it?

Chapter 2

INTERMITTENT FASTING 101

At its most basic, IF is choosing to restrict your eating. Not by dieting, or calorie-counting, or counting micros and macros, or weighing and measuring your food, but simply not eating for a predetermined amount of time. IF is a very simple concept; during a 24-hour period, one day, you choose to follow an eating pattern where you cycle between a period of eating and a period of not eating (aka clean fasting). What is clean fasting? A clean fast is when you treat yourself to one or more of five beverage choices that do not break your fast (and nothing else during your fast besides these five choices):

- black coffee, with nothing at all added to it,
- plain water, with nothing at all added to it,
- unflavored sparkling water or mineral water, like Perrier® or San Pellegrino®,
- plain black tea, with nothing at all added to it, and/or
- plain green tea, with nothing at all added to it.

One very common form of IF is called the 16/8 plan, in which you do not eat food for 16 consecutive hours (called a "clean fast"), and then eat your food and consume all of your calories (via food and beverages) within an eight-hour period of time, called an "eating window." While 16/8 is not the very best plan for losing a large amount of weight, suggested benefits of a 16/8 plan are possible weight loss, fat loss, prevention of Type 2 Diabetes, and other obesity-associated conditions ("A Guide to 16:8 Intermittent Fasting," Medical News Today Newsletter, January 17, 2020).

I advise most of my clients to start off slowly, with a very gentle 14/10 plan. This means that you would fast for 14 hours, then over the next 10 hours you would consume your calories and food for the day. Does this mean that during your 10-hour eating window you give yourself permission to graze and eat all day long, to prepare for your next 14-hour fast? No! It means that you eat two or three good meals, eat until you are satisfied and not full, and possibly a snack if you would like to have it.

Here it is in action: stop eating for the day at 8pm. From 8pm until bedtime, practice a clean fast. The reason the "clean fast" beverages don't break your fast is because none of them trigger an insulin response. When we eat and drink most beverages, our brain triggers an insulin response. As soon as that happens, your fast has been broken. Obesity is not a calorie problem, as was once thought. It is a hormone problem. Insulin is literally a fat storage hormone, and the introduction of insulin into your body breaks your fast.

When you wake up, continue with your clean fast and put off having breakfast until 10am. Voila! You have practiced a clean, 14-hour fast. You are now ready to open your 10-hour eating window. Enjoy breakfast if you love breakfast, or you can enjoy a cup of coffee with cream, or have a snack, and then have lunch and dinner. Eat enough to feel satisfied, not over-stuffed. At 8pm, you start your next 14-hour fast. Practice 14/10 for four or five days, and then slowly start building up your fasting time while shortening your eating window. Do that for four or five days, then repeat, looking something like this:

*14/10, then

*14.5/9.5, then

*15/9, then

*15.5/8.5, then

*16/8.

Although IF has many, many amazing health benefits, most people begin practicing IF for weight loss. For many people, the ideal plan for weight loss is an 18- to 20-hour fast with a 6- to 4-hour eating window. If weight loss is your goal, continue adjusting your plan until you reach:

*18/6, then 19/5, and finally 20/4. Or any combination of these three plans. Your plan does not have to be the same every single day, although until you are firmly in the habit of practicing IF every day, it is wise to keep your plan as consistent as possible.

So, the big question; what do you eat and drink during your eating window? That is 100% up to you!

IF recommends WHEN to eat, not WHAT to eat. You are totally in control of your fasting times, your window times, and your food choices when you practice IF. IF is not a diet! Will you be healthy and lose weight if you snack your way through your window, eat fast food three times a day, and have dessert every single night? Certainly not. Make the decision that you are going to do your best to eat a delicious, balanced diet. Is what you eat the primary concern when you first start practicing IF? No. Getting into the habit of practicing a clean fast every single day is the most important thing, while making healthy food choices as much as you can. When I first started practicing IF, I did still occasionally have fast food for lunch or dinner. But I greatly reduced how often I was eating fast food. I still had dessert; just not every day like I had for decades before. I made slow, sustainable changes in my food choices, and the entire time I was losing 110 pounds practicing IF, my husband and I enjoyed having Saturday night pizza night – every single week! When I was featured on the cover of Woman's World magazine in 2020, one of the things the magazine stated based on my story was that "you can do IF and eat Burger King for dinner during your first week and still lose weight!" Which was a true statement.

Yes, until you get used to IF, you may feel hunger. But the great news is that hunger isn't constant. It comes in waves. And hunger isn't harmful. The best tool for learning to consistently clean fast every single day is to stay busy!!! Have lots to do to occupy your time and your mind. Sitting around stewing about the fact that you have three more hours until you open your window will make it much harder to persist with your fast during those three hours.

Once you become "fat adapted," meaning your body has used up all of the stored glycogen in your liver (everyone has stored glycogen in their liver; this is what your body uses for fuel during your fast, until you use up all of this glycogen) and is now literally using your own body fat for fuel, you will find that your energy is greatly increased, and your hunger is greatly reduced. It takes most people between 2 to 6 weeks to become fat adapted. Being fat adapted is a goal of IF, as you want your body to burn your own body fat for fuel!

There are other forms of IF. One is called 5/2, where two non-consecutive days a week you fast all day (if desired, have one 500-calorie meal) and the other 5 days you eat normally. This is a more advanced form of fasting that I would recommend trying if you come to a plateau with weight loss using a daily IF plan. Another form of IF is to do one of the longer fasting plans, such as 19/5 or 20/4, and practice what is called OMAD, or One-Meal-A-Day, clustering all of your calories into one meal plus a snack or two if you want it, during your four- or five-hour eating window.

In my experience with IF, it took a couple of weeks for my body to adapt to this style of managing my food. The harder thing, for me, was to become adjusted to it mentally. I found it harder to wrap my brain around the fact that I was going 17, 18, 19, or 20 hours without eating.

At first, when I closed my eating window at 8pm, within an hour or two I became overwhelmed with the desire to snack, even though I had already begun my fast. So, I decided to "put myself in time-out." I would go to my bedroom for the night, to get away from food and the kitchen. I would shut and lock my door, get into my pjs, and get in bed and read, watch TV, listen to music or podcasts, or work puzzles. Anything to keep me in my bedroom, busy, and away from the kitchen! It was really hard for me at first. Mostly because it was my habit to snack in the evenings, and I was trying to break that habit. But in the morning, I felt refreshed, I was not hungry at all, and I was so incredibly proud of myself for not breaking my fast. Then, the morning was easy and the next thing I knew it was time to open my eating window. After about two weeks of practicing IF, I no longer needed to put myself in time-out at night.

IF has become wildly popular in recent years, with good reason. After I lost 110 pounds and healed several obesity and inflammation related health conditions in 14 months, my mission in life became to help others discover this amazing, healthy lifestyle. At one point, I was serving as a moderator for 12 different online IF support groups, with a combined membership of close to 500,000 members. I moderated, shared my story, encouraged others, mentored, and coached thousands of people online. I saw thousands of people, men and women, from young women all the way up to ladies in their 80s, having amazing success in losing weight and healing health issues by living an IF lifestyle.

And yet, there are still misconceptions regarding IF that persist today. I would like to address a few of these misconceptions and myths, based on my own personal experience with IF, my training as a certified health coach specializing in IF and mindset work, and the voluminous research that I have read about over the past few years related to IF.

REMINDER: before you begin any health-improvement related plan, please see your own personal physician.

<u>Myth</u>
IF is a diet.

<u>Reality</u>
IF is not a diet. It is a way to manage your food. There are no food lists, specific diets to follow, weighing and measuring food, or counting anything when you practice an IF lifestyle. However, IF works beautifully with any style of eating that you choose to practice. Or you can literally eat what you want and not practice any particular defined style of eating.

One of the hallmarks of doing IF is that over time you naturally become an intuitive eater, and you begin to crave healthier, whole, natural foods. By focusing on these types of foods, you will crowd out less healthy foods, such as processed and ultra-processed foods like cookies, cakes, pastas, and various breads. Does this mean you will never eat any of these foods? Of course not! But you will find that your tastes change, you begin to love whole, healthy foods, and these foods become what you really want to eat most of the time. When I read that this happens, I didn't believe it for a second. No way was I ever going to crave broiled fish over pizza. My opinion was that intuitive eating was the "unicorn" of the diet world – it simply didn't exist in real life! Much to my shock, this is exactly what happened to me over time as I practiced IF. When I said I was never going to diet again, I meant it. And I haven't, which still thrills me to this day.

<u>Myth</u>
You will binge and make out-of-control food choices when you break your fast.

Reality

When I first started IF, I did feel like I was eating a lot during my eating window. And research bears that out, that people do eat more after fasting…at first, and only by a few hundred calories. That certainly isn't a binge, and those few hundred calories are much fewer than you would have taken in had you been eating every few hours. I found that it didn't take more than about three weeks or so for my appetite to get adjusted to my new eating schedule, and I began to eat to match my hunger, and stop eating when I was satisfied. I was becoming aware of what it felt like to eat for health, not just out of habit or "because it was time to eat," like I had done for more than 50 years.

Myth

Fasting is starving yourself.

Reality

This is not true in the least. Fasting is making a choice to limit your eating to a certain pre-determined time period each day. Starving is not eating because you have no food; it is not a choice that anyone would make for themselves. I compare it to this. Fasting is like swimming at the beach for pleasure. Starving is like swimming to the point of utter exhaustion, to get away from a shark that you saw swimming a few feet away from you.

Myth

Fasting causes low blood sugar and shakiness.

Reality

This is a persistent myth, and nothing could be farther from the truth. As an intermittent faster, you never have to worry about your body running low on fuel to use, whether you are in your eating window or during your fast. When you start intermittent fasting, your body uses the food you are eating as fuel for up to several hours into your fast. At that point, when that food has been all used up to energize your body, your body continues to fuel you from the stored glycogen in your liver. This happens daily, until all of that stored glycogen in your liver has been used up. At that point, your body has become fat adapted. Congratulations! You eat during your window, which your body uses to fuel you until it has been used up. But now, since you don't have any more stored glycogen in your liver to fuel your body until you open your window again, your liver now breaks down your stored fat into a fuel source called ketones. Your body uses these ketones (remember, they are made from your stored fat – meaning your body is now burning your own fat) as fuel for the rest of your fast, until you open your window again. At no point during either your window or your fast is your body lacking in a fuel source; it just uses different fuel sources. Meaning no dips in blood sugar due to fasting, and no resulting shakiness.

Now, go back and read that paragraph again S-L-O-W-L-Y one sentence at a time while examining each sentence to the point of understanding it. This is a very important concept to fully understand in order to know "how" IF works for you. The more knowledge you have of how it works, the more likely you will experience a positive result.

<u>Myth</u>
Fasting will slow your metabolism.

<u>Reality</u>
While it is true that diets do slow your metabolism, IF is not a diet, and fasting has been shown to increase fat burning during the fast. Studies have shown that fasting in fact raises your basal metabolism, burning more calories than usual. When you are eating no food for a period of time, your body simply switches fuel sources, a process called being metabolically flexible, to your own body fat once you are

fat adapted. Therefore, fasting does not slow your metabolism, it increases it.

My best advice when you decide to practice an IF lifestyle? Keep it simple! Decide what plan you want to start out with, and just get started. Today. No need to wait until Monday or any other time. Eat your food during your window. When it is time to start your fast, stop eating. Period!

There are some good free fasting apps, such as *Life* and *Zero*. I highly recommend using one of them to keep track of your fasting time. They will help keep you accountable. I use *Life* and have found it to be extremely user friendly, and the act of clicking a button ensures that I remember when my fast begins and ends.

Remember that IF is not a diet. Diets usually start out easy, but the longer you are on them, the harder they get. IF starts out hard, you have to intentionally and consistently maintain your window and your clean fast – but once you become fat adapted, and the longer you practice IF, the easier it gets. It truly becomes a very easy lifestyle to maintain.

And once you become a lifetime intermittent faster, you have so many amazing health benefits to look forward to. If you told me years ago that I would lose 110 pounds and that would be the footnote to my story, I would have said you were crazy! But the physical, emotional, mental, and spiritual healing that I have experienced due to my IF lifestyle is the true headline to my story.

Chapter 3

RESET YOUR HEALTH FOR LIFE

Here is the truth. I did not begin practicing IF to lose weight, like most people do. My sister asked me if I knew about IF, which I didn't. She began to describe it to me, and I stopped her. "Hold it right there!" I said. "That sounds like some crazy fad diet. I am never going to go on a diet again, so I am not interested."

She laughed and told me it wasn't a fad or a diet, it was an ancient practice and to do my own research. IF reduces inflammation in the body and she thought it would help me with my pain issues. This got my attention! At the time, while I certainly needed to lose weight because I was back up to 249 pounds (remember: this was after my bypass surgery), my most urgent issue was that I was suffering from Achilles Tendonitis in one foot and plantar fasciitis in the other, two extremely painful foot conditions driven by obesity and inflammation. While I was still skeptical that it wasn't a diet, I was desperate to heal these painful foot conditions. So, reluctantly, I told my sister "OK, I'm going to try it. Not to lose weight, because even if I do happen to lose weight, when I quit doing IF I'll just gain it all back plus more. But I will try it to help me stop limping in pain when I walk."

My research revealed that a 19- or 20-hour fast is also an excellent plan to help promote healing in the body, so I jumped right in with a 19-hour fast. It was one of the hardest things I have ever done, and I don't recommend starting so aggressively. I only did it because I was so desperate to get out of pain. After one week, I transitioned to a 20-hour fast. After two weeks – only two weeks – my foot pain was reduced to the point that I was not limping anymore, and I was able to walk normally. I still had foot pain, but the reduction in pain was so great after just two weeks, I could walk normally. I thought this was a true miracle! So, I kept going.

After three months, since my research had revealed that longer fasting promoted even greater healing, I decided to continue with my 20/4 plan, except that I added in a 43-hour fast each week. Following this plan, after about 5 1/2 months, I was 100% pain free. I was cured of both Achilles Tendonitis and plantar fasciitis, both of which had plagued me for practically a year. Plus, as an amazing side effect, I had also lost almost 55 pounds with no dieting!

I realized that this truly wasn't a diet but an amazingly healthy lifestyle with a benefit of weight loss. Within 14 months of beginning my IF practice, I not only lost 110 pounds and healed both foot conditions, but I also resolved depression, increased my energy, eliminated brain fog, greatly improved my skin, cured my obstructive sleep apnea, and brought all of my health markers: blood pressure, cholesterol, blood glucose level, BMI, and weight, into healthy range. More miracles! Clearly practicing IF is very healing to the body, but how?

Research bears out my own experience with IF. It not only helps you lose weight; it makes you stronger and healthier. Multiple studies have shown numerous health benefits of practicing IF, from improvements in markers of heart health and blood sugar to weight loss and anti-aging effects. But how does this happen?

The first clue is the connection of insulin to our health. Research clearly shows that obesity is not a calorie problem, but it is a hormone problem. The calories in/calories out approach has been disproven and does not work. Basically, your body is always in one of two states: a fed state and a fasted state. This is true of everybody, whether you practice IF or not. During the day while you are eating (and for a few hours after), you are in a fed state. At night, while your body is not taking in any food, it is in a natural fasting state. Therefore, we call our first meal of the day breakfast, because it "breaks our fast." When you are in a fed state (and for several hours afterwards), your body releases insulin from the pancreas. You can visualize insulin as a key that opens your cells, so that the calories your body is taking in can enter your cells and your body can be fueled. With few exceptions, every time you eat or drink anything with flavors/calories, your body releases insulin. But here is the issue: insulin isn't just the key to open your cells to be able to receive and use calories to fuel your body, it also is a fat-storage hormone, putting excess calories into fat cells. Fat cannot be burned in the presence of insulin. Instead, the body uses glucose from the food you have just eaten to fuel your body instead of utilizing your fat cells.

Once your body has used up all the glucose from the food you ate to fuel your body, your insulin level falls to a very low level. With that pesky fat storage hormone insulin out of the way, your fat cells unlock and allow your body to burn fat for fuel until you eat again. Here is an easy way to think about it: you can only store more fat while you are in the fed state, and you can only burn body fat while you are in the fasted state.

This explains why it is a problem to eat every few hours, since eating and taking in calories releases insulin. All this frequent eating eventually leads to insulin resistance and Type-2 Diabetes in many people. Adding periods of abstaining from eating food, however, lets you enter the fasted state and start burning fat.

Insulin resistance has been linked to several health issues, including heart disease, stroke, high blood pressure, abdominal obesity, and many others. Putting your body into a low-insulin state by fasting on a regular basis helps lower your risk of developing these conditions.

And now we come to autophagy, another amazing natural bodily process that fasting greatly increases. Fasting has been shown to help the body repair itself, much like taking your aging car to the auto shop for new parts. Insulin has also been linked to this process. To stay healthy, your body must clean out its cells through the process of autophagy. In Greek, autophagy literally means "self-eating." Autophagy directs your body to get rid of broken down or diseased cellular components, which allows your cells to clean and renew themselves.

Here is the insulin connection: increased levels of glucose, insulin, and proteins from foods all turn OFF the process of autophagy. This explains why very frequent eating all day blocks the body from undergoing this healing process and being able to do the necessary work of cellular repair. Fasting also stimulates the body to produce human growth hormone, or HGH. HGH helps build new cells to replace the old cells that have been "eaten up" through autophagy. HGH is only released when there is no insulin present.

A classic benefit of practicing IF is lifting "brain fog." Researchers have discovered several reasons for this boost in brain function. One is the production of a protein called brain-derived neurotrophic factor (BDNF). BDNF is essential to proper brain functioning and is increased greatly during fasting. Problems with BDNF are associated with several neurodegenerative disorders, including Alzheimer's disease. BDNF promotes the growth of new neurons in a region of the brain called the hippocampus, which is involved in learning and memory, in a process called neuroplasticity. These are a lot of words to explain why researchers see great promise in reducing one's risk of developing Alzheimer's disease and other dementias by practicing IF. Both of my parents suffered from dementia and reducing my own risk of developing dementia is the biggest reason why I will always practice IF.

As I learned when I healed my own foot conditions caused by inflammation, practicing IF does reduce deadly inflammation in the body. Chronic inflammation has been linked to a long list of disorders, including arthritis, asthma, atherosclerosis, cancer, diabetes, and dementias like Alzheimer's disease. Not to mention many other conditions such as Achilles Tendonitis and plantar fasciitis. Just by reducing inflammation and producing human growth hormone (HGH), living an IF lifestyle greatly improves your odds of living longer and avoiding dementia. These are amazing benefits of living an IF lifestyle, whether you want to lose weight or not. Weight loss, stabilizing blood sugar, improving markers that produce a stronger heart and decreased stroke risk (lower blood pressure and decreases in LDL cholesterol – the bad kind of cholesterol - as well as decreased triglycerides) and increased longevity also result from practicing IF.

And, finally, non-alcoholic fatty liver disease is an obesity related condition that causes inflammation in the body. It can lead to insulin-resistance and is a risk factor for diabetes, heart attacks, and even cancer. IF has been shown in studies to reduce fat accumulation in the liver and help prevent fatty liver disease, which affects up to 25% of the U.S. population. Through my work, I have seen at least 50 people reverse their fatty liver disease through practicing IF.

We now return to the question posed at the beginning of Part I of this book…

Intermittent fasting is diet freedom: fact or fiction?

I believe you will agree with me that chapters 1-3 overwhelmingly prove that IF is, in fact, diet freedom!

PART II

ONE PAIGE AT A TIME

Chapter 4

GOAL SETTING SETS YOU FREE

One day at a time. We have all heard the expression. But how many of us take the time to reflect on what it really means? How many of us have made the decision to put this idea into practice in order to finally lose weight, achieve success in its various forms, and gain holistic health? Part II of this book is based on the concept of "one day at a time." This is how success, small wins that lead to big wins, utilizing measures of progress that encourage you, breaking free of food addiction, and achieving goals happen: one day at a time.

The goals you set can mean the difference between success and failure. The act of goal setting is creating the map for your journey. It is a mindful and intentional activity, one that requires a lot of thought. Many of us are familiar with the concept of setting a goal, but don't realize all the intricacies of setting realistic, achievable, and appropriate goals. Well-written goals should set you up for long-term success. An unrealistic goal, such as to lose 250 pounds in six months, is detrimental to your success because it is not an attainable goal. A goal of losing 60 pounds when you have a BMI (body mass index) of 19 is not an appropriate goal because it is not a healthy goal. From the world of business, we have learned of a strategy to set realistic, attainable, and appropriate goals. The acronym for this strategy is SMART goals. Specific, Measurable, Achievable, Relevant, and Timebound. What follows is how to create a SMART goal.

1. SPECIFIC: your goal should be clear and very specific, otherwise you won't be able to focus your efforts or feel very motivated to achieve it. Consider these five questions:

*What do I want to accomplish?
*Why is this goal important to me?
*Who is involved?
*Where is it located?
*Which resources or possibly limits are involved?

<u>Example</u>

My yearly physical was upsetting in 2019 when I found out that none of my health markers were in healthy range (blood pressure, cholesterol, blood glucose, weight, and BMI). This was scary because I knew that my longevity and quality of life were endangered by these poor results. My SPECIFIC goal was to improve all my health markers so that they were within the healthy range as defined by my doctor.

2. MEASURABLE: it is important for your goals to be measurable so that you can follow your progress and stay motivated. Assessing your progress as you go along helps you to stay focused, meet deadlines, and experience the excitement of making progress as you work toward your goal. Consider these questions as they relate to your goal:

*How much?
*How many?
*How will I know when my goal is accomplished?

<u>Example</u>

My MEASURABLE goal was to comply with my doctor's guidelines of checking all these health measures over the course of the next year in order to monitor progress in achieving my goal of getting all my health markers in healthy range.

3. ACHIEVABLE: your goal must be realistic and attainable to be successful. It should stretch you, but still be possible. If it doesn't stretch you, no progress will be made. If a goal is achievable, it should be able to answer these questions:

*How can I accomplish this goal?

*How realistic is my goal, based on other factors, such as time or money?

Example

I asked myself whether it was realistic to be able to shift my health markers from too high into the healthy range. I discussed with my doctor my strategy (practicing IF) to accomplish this shift to make sure my goal was realistic and ACHIEVABLE.

4. RELEVANT: this step is important to ensure that your goal matters to you and is not an idea that has been imposed on you by someone else. No matter how much your family may want you to accomplish your stated goal, if accomplishing this goal isn't really what you want, it is not relevant to you. For a goal to be relevant, we must be the one in control of achieving the goal and desiring the result. Goals get accomplished when they matter to you. If a goal is relevant, you can answer "yes" to the following questions:

*Does this seem worthwhile?

*Is this the right time for me to work on accomplishing this goal?

Example

I got honest with myself, and really considered if I was the one who wanted to get these health markers in healthy range, or if someone was pushing me to do it. It will only happen if the goal is something YOU want, not merely something someone else wants for you. After consideration, I decided that yes, this goal is relevant to me because it is my desire to shift these numbers.

5. TIMEBOUND: every goal needs a target date, so you have a deadline to focus on and something to work toward. Just saying you are going to do something with no target date invites procrastination and starting over, again and again. I know I have experienced this phenomenon many times before I started writing out my SMART goals. This part of the SMART goals criteria is designed to help prevent over-focusing on the small day-to-day tasks at the expense of accomplishing your stated goal. If you focus on eating all your food within your eating window, but don't shift your daily food choices over time, it matters not that you met the goal of eating your food within your eating window. My strategy of eating all my food within my daily eating window combined with my strategy of focusing on eating more whole, natural foods than processed foods is what helped me reach my stated goal of moving my health markers into healthy range. If a goal is time-bound, you should be able to answer these questions:

*When?
*What can I do six months from now?
*What can I do six weeks from now?
*What can I do today?

Example

Adding a time limit to shifting my health marker numbers from unhealthy to healthy was necessary for it to be time-bound. Adding "My goal is for all of my health markers to be in the healthy range in one year, at my next annual physical, as identified by my doctor" satisfied this TIMEBOUND requirement of setting a SMART goal.

Along with practicing intermittent fasting, what else did I need to do in order to meet this goal? For example, it was helpful to research suggestions for making healthy food choices, as well as exercise options, as strategies to add to my intermittent fasting toolbox. The more strategies you have available to you in your IF toolbox, the more likely you will reach your goal.

Well-planned and well-thought-out SMART goals will keep you focused and motivated. They provide a solid plan for change as you transition into a healthier lifestyle. Creating SMART goals will help protect you from overly aggressive goals which will end in disappointment. Along with creating SMART goals, there are other excellent strategies you can employ in creating goals that will help you reduce weight and improve your overall health.

There are two different types of goals: 1) Goals that focus on outcomes, and 2) goals that focus on processes. An outcome goal that I had was to lose a minimum of 100 pounds. An outcome goal focuses on what you want to achieve in the end. This type of goal is important because it gives you a target to aim for, but it doesn't address how you will achieve that goal.

Process goals are necessary to help you achieve outcome goals. For example, practice intermittent fasting daily, with a protocol of doing 18/6 – 20/4 each day was one of my process goals. It was one of the strategies I used to achieve my outcome goal. Within intermittent fasting circles, you will repeatedly hear the phrase, "Trust the process." This is exactly what trust the process means, practice fasting and eating within your window every day, take it one day at a time, and ultimately you will reach your outcome goal. Other process goals that I created were to drink water at every meal, use water to crowd out (eliminate) soft drinks, eat a certain number of fruits and veggies each day, and walking most days.

You'll notice that each of these process goals focused on actions that I took each day, one day at a time, rather than focusing on the outcome goal. The truth is that focusing on the process will ultimately determine your success! Look at it this way: if you only focus on results (achieving your final goal – your outcome goal), you will never change. If you focus on change (one day at a time, meeting your process goals), you will get results! Trusting the process helps you enjoy the journey, and before you know it you will achieve your outcome goal!

There are also long-term and short-term goals. Outcome goals are long-term goals. Many of us focus on a specific weight that we are looking to reach, or number of pounds we want to lose. But what if we thought more broadly? What if your outcome goal was a feeling – to feel confident in your own skin, or to feel truly content with what you weigh instead of continuing to reach for some unrealistic number on the scale. Or what if your outcome goal was to truly change your mindset to one that will support long-term weight loss and health, as opposed to a mindset that keeps you mired in the diet rollercoaster mentality that so many of us can't seem to escape? Some examples of short-term goals might be to fit into a specific pair of pants, to reach a certain clothing size, or to lose a small amount of weight before a special event like a wedding or a class reunion. Reaching these short-term goals goes a long way in motivating us to continue, one day at a time, to reach our outcome goals.

It is important to know that as you travel on your journey, that it is common to shift, adjust, and sometimes completely change our goals. And that is ok! With change comes growth. For example, initially my outcome goal was to cure several health conditions through intermittent fasting. I reached that goal and set a new goal to lose at least 100 pounds. As I went, though, my outcome goal changed. Much to my surprise, that number on the scale became much less important to me than my health and how I felt physically, emotionally, mentally, and spiritually. Ultimately my goal was to achieve holistic health, and to truly experience contentment and joy daily. And I reached this goal! Yes, I did lose 110 pounds, but as my priorities shifted, so did my outcome goal. Am I happy I lost the 110 pounds? Heck yes! Would I have been just as happy if I had lost 80 pounds and reached my goal of shifting my mindset and felt completely content anyway? Absolutely!

And finally, just as important as appropriate goal setting is to remember to allow for setbacks and forgive yourself when they happen.

Because we all experience setbacks. Sometimes they are small and feel manageable, and sometimes they are huge and feel like mountains that we aren't sure we are going to be able to get over. I had my own major setback after reaching the maintenance phase of my journey (see Epilogue). But because I know that IF didn't stop working, it is always there for me and it always works, and because of the mindset shifts that I experienced, I am well on my way to being back to where I feel most comfortable and content. For the first time in my life, I experienced a big weight loss setback and am still completely confident that I will rise above this challenge and get back to my health goal. I am already well on my way! This is a confidence that I have never had before, and it is one of the best benefits that I have experienced through my intermittent fasting lifestyle.

MEASURES OF SUCCESS

Let's talk about the scale! What are your feelings on it? Some folks can weigh often, even daily, with no problems at all. Other people, like myself, are not so lucky. I had a horrible relationship with the scale for most of my adult life. I let the scale have power over me. I let the scale control my feelings about myself and my mood for the day. The number on the scale was seldom where I wanted it to be, and I let this affect my confidence and my self-esteem. If I had done well on whatever diet I was on at the time the day before, I expected a loss. A big loss! And if it wasn't there, I was in a stormy mood for the day. I felt negative and discouraged and defeated. If I had a good loss, I felt jubilant. Cheated the day before? If it didn't show up yet and I still had a loss, I felt like it gave me license to cheat again today, because I got away with it. Talk about dysfunctional and unhealthy thinking. Obsessing over gains and losses, allowing an inanimate object to have control over your mood and thoughts is not the relationship I want you to have with the scale.

As a measure of success, the scale ranks poorly, for multiple reasons. Between the fluid you can gain in a day (as a result of eating and drinking and your body metabolizing nutrients) and the fluid you can lose in a day (as a result of breathing, sweating, fluid evaporating from the skin, from urine and through bowel movements), within one day there can be up to a 5 1/2-pound fluctuation, which has nothing whatsoever to do with the specific foods you ate. I know I am not alone in the psychological effect that the scale had on me.

Check this out. There is the concept of body re-composition. During fasting, the body ramps up production of human growth hormone, or HGH. HGH induces muscle building and muscle weighs heavier than fat. As we practice intermittent fasting, we are both losing fat and gaining lean muscle mass. How does this relate to the scale? We are making great progress but, on the scale, we see either no loss, or often we'll see a gain! So, while there are other measures of success than the scale, many people live and die by the scale. So, how can we make it a more reliable measure of success?

Gin Stephens, author of *Fast. Feast. Repeat.*, advises being cautious in the use of a scale to measure success, and if you choose to use it, to take specific actions to make the measure more reliable. She advises that if you are going to use the scale, that you weigh every morning. Make sure to record your weight every day. You are not going to put any stock into what the scale says on any given day, but at the end of the week, average the numbers you recorded each day for that week, and do this weekly. What you will be watching for is not a number, but the trend. Each week, is the number trending down, staying the same, or trending up? Tweak your food choices if you see that you are trending up. Trending down each week? Fantastic! Keep doing what you are doing. And if your trend line is staying the same, look at what you are doing and areas where you could improve or make better choices.

I love measuring my success in other ways besides weighing. While I do weigh occasionally to see where my weight is, there are non-scale methods that I prefer to keep track of my success. Taking measurements monthly is a great measure of success, just make sure to measure in the same spots using the same method each month. Another non-scale measure of success is to go by your clothes. How do they feel, are they getting looser, or tighter? We all really know the quality of our choices, and how our clothes fit is validation of whether we are on the right track or not. Many people like to buy a piece of clothing, such as a dress or a pair of pants. When you can barely fit into an item of clothing, then as time goes on and you try it on and it is not quite so tight, then it fits, and then gets too big, there is no greater feeling of accomplishment, in my opinion! It was so satisfying to me as I went through many sizes on my way to reaching my goal weight. One great suggestion I have is to find a great local clothing consignment store. I bought clothes that barely fit, then eventually fit, and finally got too big. I would take them back to the consignment store, sell them back, and then buy my next group of items. I went from size 22/24 to size 4/6. I had never worn sizes 4 or 6 in my life, not even when I had weight loss surgery and lost 150 pounds! At that time, the smallest size I wore was a 10. So, clearly, I am a huge fan of using clothing to measure my progress.

Another favorite non-scale measure of success that I loved as I lost weight and got healthy was to take photos each month. Make sure to wear the same outfit each time, one that is tight. Then, take photos from the front, the sides, and the back. Do this each month until that outfit gets too big. Then continue, using another outfit that is tight. Seeing yourself go down in weight in this way is thrilling!

But my very favorite way to measure my success was in NSVs, or non-scale victories. An NSV can be anything. Anything that shows progress, whether physical, emotional, mental, spiritual, etc. Any improvement in your life that is due to your intermittent fasting lifestyle can be an NSV. I kept a running list of my NSVs as I lost weight, and I am going to share it with you. I can't include every single NSV that I had as I lost weight and regained my health, but you can see the breadth and depth of things that you can and will experience as a result of living an intermittent fasting lifestyle. Your list will have NSVs on it that mine doesn't include, and my list will contain examples of NSVs that yours doesn't. And that is ok! NSVs are very personal and decided on by each of us. What is an improvement in my life and I consider an

NSV may not be something you would count as an NSV. All that matters is if you consider it an improvement based on your intermittent fasting practice.

PAIGE'S PARTIAL NON-SCALE VICTORY LIST	
I can bend over easily now and tie my shoes.	I am not super hot and sweaty all the time.
My rings fit.	My face is less puffy and my eyes are less hooded than they were.
I have healed the pain from inflammation in my feet.	I no longer have sleep apnea.
I am wearing smaller clothes sizes than ever before.	I can buy fun clothes now, and I enjoy shopping.
My depression has essentially been healed.	My confidence is much improved.
My self-esteem is much better.	I have learned to truly love myself.
My self-talk is very loving and positive now.	I have recovered from disordered, diet-brain thinking.
I have improved my general mindset and learned to see the positives in situations.	I can wear wide-calf boots from regular shoe stores again.
I have lost one shoe size.	I can find attractive clothes on sale that fit.
I have had the confidence to start my own virtual coaching business.	I can turn over in bed much easier and without pain.
I can lay on my back without pain.	I have learned not to obsess about food – I finally have food freedom!
I have my figure back.	I love to exercise now.
I have awesome energy.	I crave and love healthier foods.
I save a lot of money by not going through the fast-food drive throughs.	I got rid of my muffin top.

My thighs don't rub together anymore.

I don't avoid the stairs anymore and can climb multiple flights without getting winded.

I rarely eat for emotional reasons or for comfort anymore.

I don't have to pull myself up the stairs by the handrail anymore.

I can walk up and down the stairs without having to hold onto the handrail.

I have become an intuitive eater.

I only have clothes in my closet that fit.

I look very tone with minimal exercise.

I love my clothing size.

I love how my clothes fit.

My face isn't chubby anymore and you can see my earrings from the front.

I can now motivate and inspire others.

I can use my foot to flush the toilet in public restrooms – I could never do that before.

I feel like I have my normal personality back; I used to lack confidence to interact with others.

I now live a life gratitude.

My brain fog is gone.

I have a much more positive attitude now.

I used to quit due to slow progress; now I appreciate all progress, fast or slow.

I get compliments on my skin all the time.

I have learned to be empowered to make good health decisions for myself.

I have learned that I can trust myself, that past mistakes don't define me.

I have learned to forgive myself for slip-ups and just carry on.

Ultimately, the best measure of success is whatever works for you. Experiment and try these different suggestions. Do whatever you need to do to motivate yourself and enjoy your progress!

Chapter 6

BREAKING FREE OF FOOD ADDICTION

I began my health journey with counseling, the one thing that I had never tried before. I had always chased being skinny, but this time was different. Instead of just trying to lose weight, I wanted to get healthy and feel good about myself. It had been such a long time since I felt confident, healthy and happy. I was determined to figure out why I couldn't successfully maintain weight loss. I wanted to figure out the root cause of my issues so I could solve them once and for all. I began seeing an amazing Christian counselor.

On my first visit, I said "There is something very wrong with me. I don't know if I have a food addiction, or OCD when it comes to food and eating, or if I have an eating disorder. But whatever it is, I have got to get it figured out, because I can't continue to live this way."

I am not a mental health specialist. I was so desperate to figure out what had been happening with me for over 40 years, that I was just throwing diagnoses out there. I hesitated to use the term food addiction. Maybe, I thought, I should have said food obsession. I had heard people reference food addiction, and I was also aware that there are people who say that there is no such thing as food addiction.

I discovered intermittent fasting soon after I began counseling. With my counselor's blessing, I began to practice IF. The first few weeks were hard because I had never eaten this way before, and it was so different from eating and snacking through every day. Not long after I began counseling, the world-wide Covid shutdown occurred, and I couldn't continue with my counseling. But I kept going with intermittent fasting. And the most amazing thing happened. As I settled into my fasting routine, things changed. I became accustomed to eating in my eating window. Once I got used to fasting for 18, 19, and 20 hours at a time, and once I was fat-adapted, I no longer craved food all day. I no longer thought about food at all during my fast. I discovered that as I was losing weight, I was losing my obsession with food. What a miracle! Not only was I losing my obsession with food, but I was also losing my intense craving for sugar, sweets, desserts, and baked goods like cookies and brownies. Now, in my eating window, I truly was craving and enjoying much healthier foods. I was organically focusing on lean proteins, fruits and veggies. I still had occasional ice cream, or some other sweet treat. But they became far and few between. By then I knew that intermittent fasting was a miracle that God had brought into my life. And I absolutely believe that.

    I couldn't be in counseling long enough to have figured out exactly what my issue was. But it was clear that I didn't have OCD or an eating disorder. Neither of those conditions would have seemingly suddenly cleared up with no counseling or medication interventions. That left food addiction. Which was still confusing, because if I had a food addiction, how had it suddenly disappeared?

    So, I began to research food addiction, and what I discovered blew my mind. Have you ever wondered why it is so hard to eat just one M&M, or one potato chip? Or have you wondered why you crave sugar so badly, when you know there are much healthier options to choose from? I knew that I had loved and craved sweets for as far back as I could remember, but I just thought that was the way it was. It never occurred to me that there was a reason for it. But the answer lies in the addictive nature of sugar and salt, and in the intense and immediate gratification and pleasure they provide. In fact, sugar impacts the brain 20 times faster than nicotine, and foods that are highly processed and sweetened are the most addictive, according to Michael Moss, author of *HOOKED: Food, Free Will, and How the Food Giants Exploit Our Addictions*. Moss examined the science behind addictive foods and how they are literally engineered to trigger the brain's "on switch." You read that right. The food industry has literally spent billions of dollars over the years in search of how to make our foods as addictive as possible, in order to sell more of these foods and increase profits. It is no coincidence that "No-one can eat just one Lay's® Potato Chip!" Researchers have discovered that the crunchier and crispier our chips, cereals, and crackers are, the more we will crave them and the more we will eat. I used to wonder why, after I had already eaten two servings of my favorite caramel mini-rice cakes, I would still crave them so badly that I would go back in for more. I wasn't hungry, and intellectually I knew that there was no good reason to be eating more of them, and yet I couldn't stop myself. Imagine my shock when I discovered that this product was specifically created to make me have uncontrollable cravings for more.

In fact, many foods have a scientifically created "bliss point," a term coined by American market researcher and psychophysicist Howard Moskowitz. A food's bliss point is the exact measures of fat, sugar, and salt that optimize tastiness, make our taste buds tingle, and override the brain's natural "stop" signals. Some food items whose bliss point has been calculated include the following:

- Cakes
- Biscuits
- Doughnuts
- Ice cream
- Potato chips
- Crackers
- Muffins
- Chocolate

- Candy
- Baked goods like pastries and cookies

Bliss points have been rigorously researched and sought in order to appeal to consumer's sensory preferences. It was shocking to me that companies deliberately make food as addictive as possible. Who knew that many foods are more addictive than smoking, and the reason is because of how addictive sugar and salt are, especially when combined?

These concepts were reinforced by an incredible interview that I later came across on YouTube, entitled "How Fasting Can Reverse Aging and Prevent Disease (Fasting for Survival)." A world-renowned cardiologist, Dr. Pradip Jamnadas, MD was interviewed. The fact that a cardiologist was being interviewed surprised me but made perfect sense as I watched the video. Dr. Jamnadas explained that his priority in his practice was to practice cardiology, but his second priority was to work with his patients on their food addictions. When asked what the top three benefits of intermittent fasting were, he stated that the very top benefit of practicing IF was to cure food addiction. This interview was the first time I had ever heard that intermittent fasting cured food addiction, and yet this explained why, once I had been practicing IF for a few months, I felt like my obsession with food and particularly sugar was gone. Dr. Jamnadas detailed how the sugarier the foods are that we eat, the more we crave them. It is a vicious circle. He even went so far as to declare, "We are all, quite literally, junkies!"

Why was a cardiologist being interviewed about intermittent fasting? Because Dr. Jamnadas kept treating his patients for blockages in the arteries of their heart, and yet many of them returned six months to one year later, having developed more blockages. He examined them for risk factors for future blockages, such as smoking, Type 2 Diabetes, and high blood pressure. He found that most of these returning patients did not have these risk factors, so what was going on with these patients that caused them to develop more blockages, when other patients that he treated for blockages never had another one. On a hunch, he decided to test their insulin levels, and almost all these patients had high insulin levels. Dr. Jamnadas stated that while there was no magic pill or injection to bring insulin levels down, IF brings down insulin levels. So, this cardiologist found it necessary to treat patients' food addictions, that led to greatly increased insulin levels in the body, because high insulin levels lead to many conditions including heart attacks, strokes, and high blood pressure. This doctor literally had to work with his patients in learning to practice intermittent fasting so that he could cure their food addiction and therefore be able to treat their cardiac ailments. Shockingly, Dr. Jamnadas revealed that ultra-processed foods are connected to 11 million deaths each year. I only differ in one area from Dr. Jamnadas. He believes that patients should fix their food first, and then intermittent fast. I believe the opposite. The foundation and first priority is clean fasting, every day, with consistency. After you have your fast at the length you want it to be, THEN begin to take a look at your food choices.

I knew that intermittent fasting had somehow cured my obsession with food and my uncontrollable craving for sugar, and now I knew why. Likewise, mindful eating and eating rituals can help us slow down and think about what we eat. Research shows that the faster the addictive substances hit your brain, the more of those substances we are compelled to eat.

Lynn Rossy, author of *Savor Every Bite: Mindful Ways to Eat, Love Your Body, and Live with Joy* explains that slowing down and eating more mindfully disrupts that speed with which you eat, and therefore decreases the impact of these addictive foods. Rossy says that we can improve our relationship with food using this mindfulness approach. It is a skill that we can all learn. Being mindful of whether we are actually hungry, or if there is another reason we are eating such as being bored, longing for company and engagement, or out of stress is very important in becoming a mindful eater. Being aware of these other reasons we eat can literally help us kick food addictions.

This chapter includes information that proves that food addiction is a real thing, and that the food industry spends large amounts of money each year in learning how to keep us addicted to their products. I am thrilled to have learned that practicing an intermittent fasting lifestyle, in conjunction with practicing mindful eating, is a proven cure for food addiction. And how do those who are dealing with addictions to food, gambling, drugs, and shopping claim victory over those addictions? One day at a time!

PART III

THE NEXT PAIGE

Chapter 7

THE POWER OF HABITS

It's time to stop messing around and go deeper. Are you ready? For over 40 years, I focused solely on diets. My guess is that because you are reading this book, you totally get this. You have tried many different diets, and none have worked. That's why you're reading this. It was all about whatever diet I was doing at the time. What did that particular diet say that I should do? What should I eat? What was I not supposed to eat? How was I supposed to prepare my food? I took myself out of the equation completely and was allowing those diets to control my every move. I would do the diet to the letter, until I couldn't stand it anymore. I would lose weight, sometimes a lot! Then, when I couldn't be perfect anymore, I would quit out of frustration, and gain that weight back plus more. I never looked at my own actions and decisions, but I assigned all the blame to myself when I inevitably failed.

Then I read a quote by author James Clear that floored me. He stated, "Your current habits are perfectly designed to deliver your current results." I thought long and hard about that statement. I took time to reflect. You know how sometimes a quote or a phrase really sticks? This one did that for me. It got me thinking about my behaviors, those times when I WASN'T on a diet. The habits that I created started a long time ago, and for the first time in my life, I was looking at them for guidance. I started slowly understanding how I played a huge role in my frustrations on each diet. It wasn't really the diets. It was me!

So, I started looking at what a typical day looked like for me. I would get up and leave for work early enough to drive through a fast-food restaurant, usually McDonalds® or Hardees®, to get "breakfast" and a high calorie coffee beverage to drink during my hour-long commute. No matter what, I always got a big meal, even knowing that after I ate it, I would be stuffed. Throughout the morning, if I wasn't really busy at my desk, I would make a visit or two to the vending machine for candy or other snacks. I never made time to bring lunch, so I ate out every day. I had an hour for lunch and there were so many restaurants close by. Again, only four hours after I ate a huge breakfast and had a morning snack, I would order a large meal and eat every bite, because (like my mom told me when I was little), "You have to finish your food no matter what, because there are starving children in China." That mantra constantly played in my head. Never did an afternoon go by without me visiting the vending machine. I definitely played a huge role in the success of the multi-billion dollar vending machine companies in existence. By dinnertime, I was ready to go to another restaurant, because neither my husband nor I liked cooking. Once more, I would order a large meal and eat every bite, to the point of being so stuffed that if I opened my mouth, you could see the food sitting right there in my throat. There was no room to put any more food into my mouth, but "did someone say dessert?" There's always room for dessert, right? Monday through Friday, this was my routine every week, 52 weeks a year! And we won't even go into what weekends looked like. Whatever you can imagine, it's probably worse.

Now for the crazy part. As I reflected on what my days looked like when I wasn't on a diet, I realized there were a lot of days that I wasn't hungry at breakfast "time." I wasn't the least bit hungry in the morning. But driving through and grabbing breakfast was what I did. Just like Mr. Clear clearly stated, it was a habit I created. I realized I didn't feel a sense of control over when I ate. I just carried on with my routine each day without thought, like a zombie walking through life in a trance and not even aware of what I was doing. Heck, whether I really wanted that food or not, I was at the drive-through.

I wasn't happy with myself for doing it but, sadly, it never occurred to me that I didn't have to follow that routine. When I was on a diet, I was "good"; when I wasn't on a diet, it was a free-for-all, because of my black and white thinking. I was either all on a diet, or all off. There was no in-between. I had a real victim mentality about it. I had no understanding that this routine was my choice. It felt to me like something I did whether I wanted to or not. Can you relate? This was a routine I created decades ago, and I lived it for so many years that it seemed to be ingrained in my brain. It was just part of my life, breakfast, snacks, lunch, snacks, dinner, and more snacks. It was a bitter pill to swallow to realize that I did, in fact, create this routine. There was always choice and free will, I just didn't get it back then. I didn't order food based on hunger, I ordered food according to my routine. No wonder I always gained back what I had lost on each diet, plus more. How could I not? I ate all the time. I had zero control over my eating, I was letting food control me. Hindsight is 20/20.

In analyzing this routine through the lens of James Clear's insightful quote, I began to understand the critical importance of habits. I knew I had this ingrained routine. The definition of a routine is "a sequence of actions regularly followed," Merriam-Webster Dictionary. In other words, habits! And in my case, a series of disastrously bad habits which formed a daily routine that was detrimental to my health. And Clear was right, my habits at the time WERE perfectly designed to deliver the results I got – weight regain. It took going deeper, and looking at the power of habits, to realize that my issues went beyond just focusing on the rules of various diets.

According to James Clear in his book *Atomic Habits*, habits drive our lives and are responsible for the results we get, whether healthy or unhealthy. When I was on these various diets, I forced myself to get in the habit of following the diet's rules. I was doing it because it was what I was "supposed" to be doing. I really didn't notice that I was taking healthy daily actions by following those rules. I was only focused on following the rules (and hating them, by the way). The problem with that is that I wasn't making the decision to create specific habits for specific results. In many cases, a diet is a way to set up a process in your life, a process to learn healthy habits and incorporate them into a routine. Here is where I made a huge mistake with most of the diets I tried. I was not focusing on the process of creating healthy habits. All I could think about was following those stinking rules, and the outcome – losing weight. Does this feel familiar to you? Every day, rather than understand that by following those rules I was creating healthy habits, I just focused on results. I obsessed with my results on the scale each day. If I didn't have good losses every day, I felt like a failure. This was where my frustration came in. What I didn't know then, is if you focus on the *process* of establishing daily healthy habits, you will for sure see results down the road. Instead, I ignored the process, and only focused on *results*. That means I didn't actually create the healthy habits that the diet intended for me to, and when I eventually got tired of following all of the rules and feeling like a failure when I couldn't meet my own weight loss expectations, I would quit. Again! I totally missed the point.

    I'd like you to take a minute to think of something you do on a regular basis without thought. A habit that you created out of repetition. Go ahead and write it right here in the book (if you're reading the print version) or on a piece of paper (if you're reading the digital version). Then think about how that action affects your life. Is it really a habit? Is it something you do mindlessly? A habit that was created from past experience? A habit that was created when you were young and you've "just done your whole life"?

It was not until I began practicing intermittent fasting that I came to understand the distinction between focusing on the process rather than focusing on results. Among seasoned intermittent fasters, one phrase you will repeatedly hear is "Trust the process!" It took me awhile to figure out what that really meant, but trusting the process is actually a life-saving action. When people ask me what I did differently this time, to be able to lose 110 pounds instead of flounder unsuccessfully and then quickly quit, this was key. "The process" is just forming a series of healthy habits! Practicing intermittent fasting, with its daily eating window and clean fast, is a set of healthy habits that formed a new routine for me to follow. Within the framework of a routine being a series of habits, it was comforting for me to have a routine that I focused on and followed every day. I learned to quit worrying about the scale and weight loss, and to just follow that routine, no matter what. By focusing on my routine every day, before I knew it, I began having fantastic results!

In fact, please don't miss the critical importance of habits. The whole issue of trusting the process and realizing that habits are so influential in directing our lives really ignited my curiosity about forming healthy habits. How does that happen? I had no clue, and yet I realized that I had inadvertently discovered something that had been missing for me all those years of yo-yo dieting and morbid obesity that I had endured.

Much of the game-changing information I learned about the importance of habits and routines came from *Atomic Habits*. Clear describes habits as behavioral patterns that shape who we are. The beauty of habits is that we can decide to utilize the power of habits to guide our lives in a healthy, positive way. The goal in using habits to affect our health outcomes is to take a specific action every day, consistently, until it becomes automatic. When is the last time you got ready for work and considered whether you felt like brushing your teeth or not?

Or got in the shower and pondered whether you were in the mood to wash your body or not? These actions are habits that are ingrained in us from doing them consistently over time. The goal is to identify actions that, when practiced consistently, become second nature. Habits take away our need to make decisions. Decision-making and habits are opposites. Once something is a habit, you are free from having to decide to do the right thing. Habits require no thought or willpower at all. They save us from being bombarded each day with a multitude of decisions like whether to brush our teeth, take out the trash when the trash can is full, exercise, make healthy food choices, or practice self-care. Once these actions become habits, they become "just what you do." In developing habits, repetition and consistency are key.

A great example of a routine being an accumulation of habits is your commute to work. You don't give it a second thought to buckle your seat belt, you just do it. Your hand places the key in the ignition, or you push the start button, without your deciding to do so. Checking your blind spots as you pull out of the driveway, or your parking spot, are second nature. And aren't you glad they are? How cumbersome would it be if you had to actively think and decide to take each of these actions? And this is just one small example made up of one daily routine!

If you want to start a new habit, there is no way around the fact that to make it an ingrained habit you must repeat the behavior over and over until it becomes automatic, at which point you do it without having to exert willpower to make yourself do it. Willpower and/or motivation may get you started, but habit is what will keep you going.

This was my experience when I decided to start intermittent fasting, which, as it turns out, was the first healthy routine, made up of good habits, that I established on my journey. It was definitely a new behavior to skip breakfast. It was hard because it had been my habit to have a big breakfast every day. I decided, in fact, that it was just too hard for me to go "cold turkey" and yet I didn't want to break my fast. So, I decided to "have breakfast." Each day, I sat at the kitchen table and had an iced black coffee. This was my breakfast. I did it every day. At that time, I hadn't yet learned the information about habits and routines, I just instinctively knew I had to replace the act of having breakfast with some other specific act. And it was so helpful! I had to get used to waiting to eat until my window opened. There was no other way around it. I had to do the hard work of making myself wait. I did that by keeping very busy and trying not to focus on eating. It took time and patience. It didn't come automatically, I had to do the work necessary to practice these behaviors every single day. I had to get used to eating normally within my eating window. At first, I ate too much, because my mind was telling me I was starving since I had fasted. And the reality is that in the first few weeks of starting intermittent fasting, you might get hungry. Again, every day I did my best to eat normally within my eating window. Day after day after day I took these same actions. I had my iced coffee for breakfast. I held on until time to open my window. I ate my food within my window and closed my window when it was time. It took about two weeks to really begin to feel comfortable with this new routine. Not long after that, it became totally ingrained and became easy. This was my new routine and I loved it, because I felt great, and knew I was doing something healthy and amazing for my body. Slowly I learned that valuable lesson, to focus on the process, not the result.

Going from eating practically every minute of every day to moving into a place of intermittent fasting didn't happen overnight. Those three weeks or so before I was fully immersed enough that my cravings were gone took work. But at that point, I no longer went through the drive-through. With that said, I still occasionally go through the drive-through, but I don't order as much food as I used to, I make different choices most of the time, and I don't do it outside of my eating window.

When I am fasting, I steer clear of the drive-through, the walk-in, any kind of food. And I don't even have to think about it; I don't have to decide if I am going to eat anything during my fasting time. Why? Because I developed a series of healthy habits that created a new routine for me, a routine that became second nature and took away decision-making. This routine allowed me to be IN CONTROL, and that is a gift beyond measure. And all because I decided to trust the process, and I learned critical information on habits. This life-changing information of how to develop routines and healthy habits is one of THE biggest reasons that I was finally able to be successful in losing weight and regaining my health.

Chapter 8

GOOD HABITS CHANGED MY STORY

Diving deeper into habit change showed me that the power of habits can help us lead healthy lives and even prolong our lives. Starting with the outcomes you want, you can identify specific habits that will help you reach your desired outcomes. Quite literally the good habits that I developed changed my story, and the same can happen for you. Soon after I began practicing intermittent fasting, I began reading about habit change and understanding how habits drive our lives. I came to understand that developing healthy habits requires intention, specific action, repetition, and patience. Above all, I learned that consistency is critical in developing new habits. Consistency is the one thing that can overcome any obstacle, such as plateaus or occasional overindulgences. No matter how slowly you may be losing weight, if you are consistently practicing your healthy habits and routines each day, you will be successful. It is also very helpful to have specific strategies to develop good habits.

Make it Easy by Controlling Your Environment

When you are starting a new habit, there is nothing to be gained by trying to do something really hard all at once. It is challenging enough to establish healthy habits, one thing you can do to encourage success is to make it as easy as possible. One strategy to make it easy is to control your environment. This really is a specific strategy, and much to my delight it really works.

I decided to make it as easy as possible on myself to make good food choices in my eating window. I did that by controlling the environment in my kitchen. I quit buying lots of sweets and sugary treats. I quit buying candy for the house. I stopped buying lots of ultra-processed foods to have in the pantry. I figured if isn't in the kitchen, I can't eat it. Or at least, not without going to the trouble to get out at night to go and get something I might be craving. It just wasn't worth the effort. I started buying my favorite fruits to have as snacks and dessert. I shopped the perimeter of the grocery store to focus on whole foods without barcodes. All those ultra-processed foods are housed on the inner isles of the grocery store. Fresh fruits, vegetables and protein from the butcher counter don't have barcodes. I focused on buying these kinds of foods. And I did not deprive myself of occasional treats; this was key when I first started intermittent fasting. But when I did want a dessert or treat, I would go out and get a single serve portion, like going to an ice cream parlor for one scoop of ice cream to enjoy rather than keeping a gallon in the freezer.

Another way that I controlled my environment and made it easy when I first started intermittent fasting was to "put myself in time-out" in the evenings. I was used to snacking at night and at first this was my hardest time of the day. Clean fasting was a tough sell to a girl who loved her evening snacks! So, after I had closed my window, when I began wanting a snack so badly, I could literally taste it, I decided to make things easy on myself. I would get away from the kitchen by going upstairs to my bedroom. I would shut and lock my bedroom door, get into my pajamas, and spend the evening in my room. I would occupy myself by reading, watching TV, listening to music, doing crossword puzzles, talking to friends or family on the phone, or listening to podcasts, which was one of my favorite things to do. There are a lot of great podcasts that focus on intermittent fasting and success stories. I did whatever I had to do to stay in my bedroom for the evening. In the morning, I felt fantastic. I wasn't hungry at all, felt so proud of myself that I had maintained my clean fast, and it got my day off to a great start. I regularly put myself in time-out for about two weeks, the length of time that it took for those nighttime cravings to diminish. At the end of two weeks, I had gotten used to clean fasting in the evening. It had become easy not to go into the kitchen and grab a snack and I no longer needed my hack of putting myself in time-out. I had controlled my environment and made it easy for myself.

Take Tiny Steps, and Make it Enjoyable

These strategies worked especially well for me when I was at the point in my journey that I felt drawn to starting an exercise program. When I had lost about 60 pounds and wanted to begin walking, I knew I had to find some way to make it fun or enjoyable, because it had been a long time since I last walked for exercise. Also, since one mistake I had repeatedly made in the past was to start with too much exercise, too soon, leading me to quit quickly, I decided to start small. I made a rule for myself that I would walk most days, but only for 20 minutes. Could I have done more? Of course! But at first I wasn't really getting into the habit of walking. I was getting into a routine of getting up every morning, putting on my walking shoes, and hitting the pavement. That routine, made up of three individual habits, was my segue into walking. To make it something that I looked forward to rather than dreading, I decided to always take my iPhone with my awesome playlist on it, and my wireless earbuds, and listen to the music that I love – every time I walked. Honestly, I didn't start out loving walking. I chose to walk because I wanted to get in better physical shape, but listening to music was what I looked forward to. For quite a while walking was just what I did every morning while I enjoyed listening to my extensive playlist. I gradually added time and distance to my walk. Before I knew it, not only was I equally loving walking and listening to music, but I had worked my way up to being a fitness walker, walking 3 to 6 miles, at 15 to 15 1/2-minute miles, most days. And loving it! Not bad for a 57-year-old, I thought! I got in the best shape of my life, between fast walking and intermittent fasting, and all because I made the decision to incorporate walking as a daily habit. Pairing a habit that wasn't especially enticing with an activity that I really enjoyed, was a fantastic strategy to help me become a walker. The lesson that I had learned about focusing on the process (only focusing on enjoying walking and listening to music every day), rather than the outcome (wanting to be in great shape too quickly) served me well once again.

Taking very small steps, often called micro steps, is often the key to building a successful healthy habit. In building my walking habit, I started out doing much less than I knew I could. But I wanted it to be quick and easy starting out. If one day I wanted to do more than 20 minutes that was fine, but if I didn't, I could still feel very successful because I had achieved my goal of walking for 20 minutes. The strategy of taking a very small action, such as meditating for five minutes every day and building up more time from there works! The goal is not to overwhelm yourself starting out, and very slowly build up. If I want to enter a competition to see who could do the most planks, I would start with doing one plank a day. Then I would build to doing two planks a day, and slowly work my way up to competition level.

Choose the Identity You Want to Have

For all those years I was stuck in the yo-yo diet rut, I felt like a failure. I thought of myself as a lazy, unmotivated fat woman. There, I said it, and it wasn't easy to share. But it is true. I felt like a person who could never accomplish a goal. I felt like a loser, a quitter. This was the identity that I had for so many years. No, it wasn't an identity that I chose or wanted. It was an identity that I developed based on my choices and behaviors – in other words, my habits. Remember when I said that habits drive our lives? This is what I allowed to happen to me. I created horribly bad habits. I had routines around eating and food choices that were very bad for me, both physically and mentally. James Clear says that the quickest way to change what you do is to change who you want to be. All those years my identity was formed because of my habits and the resulting feelings they caused. But if we choose a different identity, you can bet we will work hard to build new habits that support that identity.

For example, I identify as a writer. I become a writer by writing every day. Writing every day is a habit consistent with being a writer. Or what if I wanted to identify as a long-distance runner. I would develop habits that would be consistent with being a long-distance runner, such as getting up every morning, putting on my exercise clothes and running shoes, and getting out and running consistently longer and longer distances. You can change your habits to match who you want to be.

Along the way, I was surprised to find that I developed an identity as a walker. I thought of myself as a walker, so I made sure I walked almost every day. By walking, I reinforced my identity as a walker. I developed an identity as an intermittent faster. Again, by clean fasting every day and eating within my eating window only, I reinforced the identity of an intermittent faster. Eventually, I developed an identity as a fit, healthy woman, so I worked as hard as I could to take actions every day that supported that identity.

I had never felt these things before. I was able to develop this identity because I built habits consistent with being a fit, healthy woman. I took actions that a fit woman would take, such as intermittent fasting and walking, not a woman who was a lazy person who avoided exercise and healthy food choices like the plague. Deciding who you want to be is one of the best ways to change your actions and develop healthy new habits and routines.

Create a Ritual

Another way to build a healthy habit is to create a special ritual around that habit. When I wanted to start drinking more water every day, I elevated the act of drinking water by purchasing a large, attractive floral water tumbler that keeps my water ice cold. I created a ritual of only using that tumbler to drink water. I fill it with ice water, drink all of it, then refill it as I empty it. I drink three of these every single day. Filling my tumbler with ice water is the first thing I do every day when I come downstairs. By ritualizing the act of drinking water from a special container, drinking water feels like an action to savor and value more. It feels important. Research published in *Psychological Science* tested whether rituals around food, such as swirling wine in a glass before drinking it or stirring your tea and clinking the spoon on the side, make us savor foods more. This is precisely what the scientists found does happen, based on a series of experiments.

Here's another example of creating a ritual: I wanted to get more sleep so that I felt more awake during the day, because I make better food choices when I'm not exhausted. Therefore, I had to figure out a way to make going to bed happen easily. I often dread bedtime because bedtime isn't just getting in bed. It is brushing and flossing my teeth, washing my face, putting moisturizer on my face, neck and hands, and getting into my pjs. Going to bed involves a lot of time-consuming actions that I don't look forward to. Therefore, I dreaded and put off bedtime. So, I decided to create a new ritual. I set my new bedtime at 10:30pm. At least an hour before bedtime, I started going up to my bathroom and doing all the 'pre-bedtime' preparation so that when bedtime came, literally all I had to do was get in bed. This ritual of getting ready for bed early made such a huge difference. It made going to bed at the time I wanted easy.

Here's the thing. To develop all these healthy habits, I had to do the work. I had to plan and take consistent action every day to make these actions ingrained habits. And the truth is that with healthy habits, you must take small, intentional steps to achieve that habit. Why are we discussing all these various strategies in a chapter focused on good habits? Because they are the habits that take work! When I was in the habit of driving through and getting a big breakfast every morning, that was a bad habit – and it was easy. It did not require planning, micro steps, looking for some way to make that action enjoyable. It was all too easy to drive through and get a big, delicious breakfast. Bad habits are easy. We fall into them. They do not require any effort to develop. They are pleasurable in the moment, but detrimental in the long run. We don't just happen to fall into healthy habits. You will never just drift toward a healthy habit. So, let's look at some healthy habits that will help you reach your goal of a long and healthy life. These are some of the healthy habits that I developed over time, and they helped me to finally be able to lose weight successfully!

- Practice intermittent fasting daily.
- Practice a clean fast daily.
- Choose natural, whole food options 80% of the time for their deliciousness and health; choose a treat 20% of the time, for fun and enjoyment and delight.
- Establish a consistent routine during your window; for example, enjoy two meals and one snack, or eat one meal and a couple of snacks, called OMAD (One Meal a Day).
- When you begin your intermittent fasting lifestyle, choose a protocol you want based on your goals, and work your way up to that. Then, stick with that protocol consistently.
- Once your protocol is established so that it is second nature, vary it occasionally. Variety is good for your body. One day do 18/6, the next day do 20/4, another day do 16/8, etc.

- It is great for your gut health to eat a variety of foods like various protein sources, a variety of fruits, more than just a couple of kinds of vegetables, etc. Avoid eating the same thing day in and day out.
- Get in healthy movement that you enjoy most days.
- Develop a habit of gratitude. Why? It will make you feel happy, and happiness is good for you!
- Focus on the process, not the result. If you focus on what you do every day, your habits and choices, you will certainly have a good outcome down the road. If you only focus on daily results, you will be anxious and won't make the necessary changes to develop good habits.

Identify something YOU want to develop as a healthy habit based on your needs and goals. Then do that thing with repetition and consistency until it becomes second nature and you don't have to think about doing it. Until it becomes automatic. Then choose another one, and so on.

Chapter 9

BAD BEHAVIORS BREAKDOWN

Ahhh, our bad behaviors. We have a love/hate relationship with them, don't we? Remember, bad behaviors are easy to fall into. Who has to develop strategies to sit around and watch TV all day? Or eat practically a whole bag of chips? We know they are bad, and yet in the moment they feel so good. It is so enjoyable to eat that pint of ice cream with a spoon, right out of the container, at the end of a stressful day. But while they feel good in the moment, they can make us feel bad about ourselves later. These bad behaviors start so easily, yet are so challenging to stop.

But what are behaviors (either good or bad) repeated consistently? They are habits! So let's call them what they are, bad habits. One thing I learned through my experience of yo-yo dieting for over 40 years is that either you choose your habits based on the outcomes you want, or your habits will choose you and give you outcomes that you would never want. Bad habits take you further away from your goals. Fortunately, just as strategies can be utilized to create good habits, strategies can be used to eliminate bad habits.

Attack the Swarm to Succeed

One of the most successful strategies I found to eliminate bad habits came from another fantastic book, *Tiny Habits*, by BJ Fogg, Ph.D. Fogg states that when we think of a bad habit that we need to eliminate, most of the time it is a general habit that is made up of lots of bad habits. This group of bad habits is called the Swarm. This strategy involves identifying a general habit, and then underneath of it, write all the individual bad habits that together make up the general habit. Here was my first attempt to utilize this strategy. The general habit that I identified was bad eating habits. Underneath my general habit, you will see the Swarm of habits that together make up the general habit of bad eating habits.

Bad Eating Habits

- Grazing and snacking all day.
- Avoiding fruits, vegetables, and other whole natural foods.
- Eating lots of sugary foods and lots of processed carbs.
- Loading my diet with ultra-processed foods like cakes, crackers, pasta, and rice.
- Eating until I was Thanksgiving stuffed at practically every meal.
- Drinking calories in beverages such as fruit juices, diet soft drinks, and alcohol rather than eating good, nutritious, satisfying whole fruits and foods.
- Eating lots of fast food with few nutrients.

Once I identified the Swarm, my first task was to pick the easiest bad habit to eliminate. Since I had become an intermittent faster, by default I had already stopped grazing and snacking all day. Done! Since that habit had already been eliminated, I was ready to go on to the next habit that would be easiest to get rid of. The next one I chose was to stop drinking calories rather than eating them in foods. This didn't seem to be too hard at first, because fruit juices and alcohol were easy for me to give up within my window. Harder, though, was diet soft drinks. Even though they weren't loaded with calories like the other drinks were, I had heard for years that they are worse for you than regular soft drinks. This seemed like a great time to stop drinking them. So, I stopped drinking them cold turkey. Boy, that was much harder than I expected!

I focused on drinking water and tea during my window. I ignored my cravings, and essentially white-knuckled it. After one month, a day came when I was just positive that I was going to die if I didn't have a Diet Coke®, right that minute! So, I made an excuse to myself and said, "Oh, one Diet Coke® isn't going to kill you." I got a medium Diet Coke® from a drive-through, took one drink and almost spat it out. It tasted horrible. All I could taste was an awful chemical taste. I threw away the rest of it and didn't have those cravings anymore. When you try this strategy, BJ Fogg has a whole list of micro-strategies to eliminate bad habits that are especially challenging that you can try, in case you don't want to try the cold turkey method.

One at a time, I tackled each of the bad habits in the Swarm. And, one-by-one, I eliminated them. It took time, persistence, hard work and patience. But the effort was so worth it. I felt so successful that I decided to get brave and identify another general habit that I wanted to eliminate. This time I identified bad exercise habits. Below you will see the Swarm of habits that I identified.

Bad Exercise Habits

- ➢ Doing too much, too fast.
- ➢ Being a weekend warrior and injuring myself, rather than building up slowly and safely.
- ➢ Failing to stretch.
- ➢ Buying gym memberships and exercise equipment, then not using them.

- Doing exercise that I hate rather than incorporating movement that I like.
- Not being consistent with exercise.
- Only doing cardio and ignoring resistance training.
- Not doing resistance training safely.

I have already described my experience with beginning my exercise program. This was how I started. The easiest thing to eliminate first was to stop joining gyms and buying exercise equipment that I never used. I eliminated doing too much, too fast by starting out "tiny," as BJ Fogg recommends. Each time something from the Swarm was eliminated, I felt accomplished and proud and that gave me great momentum going forward and tackling other bad habits in the Swarm. I highly recommend you try this strategy to get rid of your bad habits. In fact, right now, go ahead and identify a general bad habit, and then tease out the bad habits that make up the Swarm for that general habit. You won't believe how helpful this exercise is, and how motivating it is each time you eliminate a bad habit from the Swarm.

(General Bad Habit)

- _____
- _____
- _____
- _____
- _____
- _____

Choose the easiest bad habit in the Swarm to eliminate first, then email me at fastinwithpaige@gmail.com and tell me what your Swarm is for this habit. I truly want to know. Take pride in succeeding. Then, move on to the next easiest, and so on. Take as long as you need on each one and build on your success. Don't forget that as they become more challenging to eliminate, try the micro-strategies from *Tiny Habits* to help you. Both *Atomic Habits* and *Tiny Habits* are available at your local public library. It was helpful for me to check both out. They were amazing resources for me, and they will be for you as well.

Reward Yourself

Reward yourself for eliminating bad habits. Who doesn't love a great reward, and in fact using rewards is a great way to influence behavior. I tried this strategy when I decided that I was drinking way too many high-calorie coffee beverages in my window. Oh, who am I kidding? They were glorified milkshakes posing as coffee. Even though I only had them in my eating window, I certainly wasn't doing myself any favors, and I found myself having them more and more often. Just because you can do something, doesn't mean you should.

So, I set up a jar labeled "New Boots." I had seen an expensive pair of boots that I really wanted and decided that each time I passed on getting one of those coffee drinks, I would add $5 (the cost of my high-calorie coffee beverage) to my New Boots jar. It motivated me and helped me get rid of that bad habit. By the time I had enough money to purchase the boots, I had eliminated the habit. You can adapt this strategy to lots of different situations, and bad habits that you want to eliminate. Make sure the reward is something special, something you really want.

Peer Modeling

At one point, as I was losing weight, I asked a close friend of mine if he had any strategies that he liked to use to eliminate bad habits. He is a disciplined guy and has lifted weights with a lifting partner three times a week for many years, without fail. He works at a gym and sees lots of people who have lost weight and who really inspired him. Mark said he sees clients all the time who never eat carbs, who have completely cut out sugar, and never miss their days at the gym. He had found himself weighing 281, an all-time high weight for him. He was drawn to the idea of eliminating sugar like a few of his gym buddies had done, but he felt that total elimination wasn't exactly appealing. So, he decided to break it down, and do part of what they had done. He figured it sure couldn't hurt and at least would be a good start. So, he decided to limit sugar to once a week, on Saturday, with a meal. Mark started this regimen August 1, 2021. It was slow going. Not a lot happened it seemed. But he stuck with it. He consistently avoided sugar all week and allowed himself one treat on Saturdays with a meal. Mark's persistence and repetition paid off. He has now lost 40 pounds, eight months after starting his plan of having something with sugar only once a week. He said it was occasionally hard and there were evenings he would have enjoyed a brownie or some ice cream, but he remained strong. He didn't make any other changes to his diet; he eats twice per day, eats what he wants, and is happy with his food choices. He is thrilled with his progress and feels great.

I loved the idea of peer modeling. Looking to what a friend or family member has done and modeling their behavior relative to a goal that you want to accomplish, or in this case, to eliminate a bad habit. It is very wellestablished that those you spend time with have a direct impact on the choices you make, including your food choices. We tend to want to feel included and a part of things, and we often prefer not to feel different. In *Atomic Habits*, James Clear says that peer pressure is only bad if you are surrounded by bad influences. He further shares that he often imitates the behavior of those around him without realizing it. Peer modeling is a great way to get ideas on how to eliminate bad habits, when you see a peer, friend or family member accomplish something that you would like to accomplish. Be sure to utilize the power of peers in your life to get fresh ideas on how to succeed.

Another very similar idea to peer modeling is to choose an accountability buddy. This accountability relationship has seen many people succeed in eliminating bad habits because of the support and accountability they receive. I have a fantastic accountability buddy. She inspires me and supports me and encourages me when I fall short of my goals. She tells it like it is and is very wise. We have an informal relationship where we text each other, if not every single day every other day or so. Some people choose an accountability buddy and formalize the relationship. One way to do this is to draw up a written contract that states what you will do, what you will stop doing, and when. Such contracts have even been written that include negative consequences that will happen if you don't accomplish your goals by the identified date. This document is signed by both parties. Personally, a written contract isn't my cup of tea. But who knows, it could be right up your alley. The great thing is that it is between you and your accountability buddy what kind of relationship you want to have. Keep in mind that many people find that the relationship with an accountability buddy has helped them in feeling supported as they eliminate bad habits. It is an idea to try, and the more ideas and strategies that you have in your intermittent fasting toolkit as you work to eliminate bad habits, the better!

Make it Invisible

This strategy to eliminate a bad habit may seem obvious, but it bears mentioning – because it is effective. If you have a favorite dessert at a particular restaurant, and you are accustomed to having that dessert every single time you go to that restaurant, you can make that dessert invisible. Do not go to that restaurant. If you aren't there, if you don't see it, you won't order and eat it. This concept is like controlling your environment. If you always sit in a particular chair every night and munch on chips, sit on the couch and do not ever snack when you are sitting on the couch. If going to the movies always involves a large popcorn, candy and a large soda, stream movies and stay away from the movie theater. Some may say this is cheating, but every advantage you can give yourself is a bonus. Your goal is to eliminate those bad habits that have been hanging around for years, so utilize every single strategy you can. The effort will always be worth it and will pay off in improved health and longevity for you.

PART IV

PAIGE TURNER

Chapter 10

SELF-LOVE & SELF-CARE

It is time to turn our focus to some critical issues, the really deep ones. Self-love and self-care, the influence of mindset on our health and weight loss journey, and healthy movement for our bodies. Why did I save this information for last?

I have gone over the basics of intermittent fasting and how it will heal your body and soul in Chapters 1 through 3. I talked about how important it is to set goals, and how to break food addiction with intermittent fasting in Chapters 4 through 6. And I have shared vital information about the power of habits and how they can either dictate our success or be our downfall in Chapters 7 through 9. But now it is time to literally turn the page in the creation of your new, successful story. In all those years that I was never successful in my many weight loss attempts, it turns out that the subjects we will discuss in Part IV are the essential, but elusive, pieces to the puzzle of successfully losing weight and keeping it off. These were the puzzle pieces that I was missing. They are what the surgeon was referring to when he said he could operate on my stomach, but not my brain. I am one of the biggest proponents of intermittent fasting on the planet. It is an amazing vehicle to change our lives and our health status. I will always be an intermittent faster for the amazing health benefits, longevity, and disease prevention that it offers. But I am here to tell you that if you don't take the information in Part IV very seriously and make real changes in your life in these areas, your ability to have success with sustainable weight loss and making health gains will be greatly diminished. That is how important this information is, and I really want you to Turn the Paige in making YOUR story a success story!

Do you know what it means to love yourself? Doesn't everyone automatically love themselves? If asked, most people would say, "Of course I love myself." What would YOU say, and do your actions reflect true self-love?

I used to hear people say, "You have to love yourself" or you have to "Love yourself first." Frankly, I always thought that was just a silly thing to say. Of course I love myself. Who doesn't love themselves? As it turns out, the joke was on me. For too many years my actions and thoughts certainly did not reflect love for myself. I ate terribly unhealthy foods daily. I didn't get enough sleep, ever. I got very little healthy movement; in fact, I was a true couch potato. After work I would be so tired, I would spend every evening with a snack in front of the TV, and weekends were made for relaxing, snacking, and TV… or so I thought. I didn't purchase fun, cute clothes that made me feel confident. I thought I had to wait until I finally lost weight to dress fashionably. What was I waiting for? Sadly, I did not recognize that life itself is a special occasion and that I deserved to be nurtured. Self-love was clearly not in my vocabulary, but it is now. Back then, I had no clue what it really meant to love yourself. I just thought it was a given. A feeling. Little did I know that thoughts and actions demonstrate self-love, and clearly none of my thoughts or actions did that. How do we love ourselves, and why does it matter? What does true self-love mean to you?

The definition of self-love is that you accept yourself fully, treat yourself with kindness and respect, and nurture your own growth and well-being. It encompasses not only how you treat yourself, but also your thoughts and feelings about yourself. When you think about self-love, you can imagine what you would do for yourself, how you would talk to yourself, and how you would feel about yourself that reflects love and concern. When you love yourself, you have an overall positive view of yourself. It doesn't mean you feel positive about yourself all the time, though. That wouldn't even be realistic. For example, I can temporarily feel upset, mad, or disappointed in myself, just like you can occasionally feel about other people you love. But those feelings are temporary and never mean that you don't love that person anymore. While you are feeling those feelings, your love for that person directs how you relate to them, get over being mad or disappointed in them, and forgive them. You can do these things specifically because you DO love them. And the same goes for you. You love yourself just like you love your family and close friends. You deserve to feel amazing and confident. Loving yourself is recognizing that you are a wonderful person right now, just as you are. Your worth is not determined by your size. You are a complex, interesting, vibrant person with countless positive attributes and people who love you. Today. No matter your size. I have heard it said that if you don't love yourself, you can't truly love others, because you have not really experienced love. I believe this to be true.

Wow, I just did a deep dive into exactly what self-love means. I did it because I figured that if I had no clue what it truly means to love yourself, you might not know either. I wanted to make it crystal clear what it means, because until you truly do love yourself, you won't be successful long-term in your weight loss and health efforts. The bottom line is that loving yourself, and I mean truly loving yourself as described above, is a key piece of that puzzle of successful weight loss and attaining great health, joy, and contentment in your life.

It wasn't until I was in my 50s that I first became aware of how horribly I talked to and treated myself. What was my first clue that I truly didn't love myself? I talked to myself in a way that I would never ever talk to any other person, not even my worst enemy. I was mean to myself, and very negative with myself, <u>all the time</u>. I never acknowledged any good things I did, but I sure went overboard chastising myself for any mistakes that I made. I told myself I was a failure, that I would never lose weight for good because I had no willpower, I had always been a failure at trying to lose weight and I was never going to change. When I was doing those aforementioned diets, when I couldn't be perfect (and who could ever be perfect), I would beat myself up, told myself how I had messed up yet again, and that I might as well give up. Because I had been talking to myself this way since I was a young teenager, I didn't even realize what I was doing. This self-deprecating personality trait started developing at approximately age 10 and continued until 56. That's 46 years of baggage I needed to turn around. I could go on and on repeating the terrible things I said to myself, but you get the picture. And to make it worse, I believed all these things I told myself. My self-esteem and confidence were terribly low. How could they not be in the face of this constant barrage of negativity and cruelty that I directed at myself? I was my own worst bully.

Thinking about the information that you just read about self-love, you can see that I clearly didn't love myself. Our thoughts and words to ourselves demonstrate our self-love or lack of it. All those mean thoughts about myself? I just thought that was the way it was. That it was WHO I was. What I have learned is that we believe what we tell ourselves, whether it is true or not, whether it is negative or positive.

The other thing I learned was that negative self-talk is the very worst habit of all, the most devastating to our ability to love ourselves and, thus, the reason we will never be successful with our weight loss and health improvement attempts if we don't turn it around. It is imperative and possible to change your self-talk no matter your age. This negative, harsh, and punitive self-talk is the number one reason that for over 40 years I failed to lose weight and keep it off. Awareness is the first step in healing and my awareness at age 56 was instrumental in my actions from that point forward. You certainly can't correct something that you aren't aware of. I realized that I had been telling myself things for years that weren't true, but were born out of sad, negative emotions as a child. I understood that if this was a bad habit, there must be some way to turn it around and become my own best friend and cheerleader. I intuitively knew that until I corrected this horrible habit, I would never really be able to love myself. This negative self-talk "HABIT" was keeping me from loving myself. But how? I had no clue how to turn this around. Negativity came naturally to me and was deeply ingrained in my brain. It was automatic. Thinking about what I had learned about habit change, I knew that I had to break this damaging habit. I knew I had to change my thoughts, but wow, what a daunting task. After lots of thought and prayer about it, I came up with a plan to 'halt the talk.' If you are aware that negative self-talk is an issue for you and you're ready to stop being your own bully and turn into your own best friend, I am going to share how I solved this problem and how you can, too.

I want you to become hyper aware of how you talk to yourself. You are going to monitor your self-talk very closely. Every time you catch yourself engaging in self-talk that is punitive, mean, impatient, unforgiving, critical, or just plain hateful, follow the steps that I am going to outline below. Every. Single. Time! This takes intentional practice, patience, persistence, and consistency. It takes time because change doesn't happen overnight. Keep following these steps, though, and over time, you will find that your negative self-talk has become positive, loving, gentle and kind. You will learn to love yourself enough to treat yourself with respect and to give yourself grace. Bear in mind that eliminating negative and mean self-talk is the first step in learning how to demonstrate that you love yourself.

1. When you realize you are talking terribly to yourself, immediately say STOP! to yourself. Literally. Either in your head, or

out loud. Even if you feel silly, do it. Do not skip this step because you think it sounds silly! This is a crucial first step.

2. Think of a person that you love with all your heart. It could be a parent, sibling, child, or friend. It must be someone that you would never speak to in the way that you speak to yourself.

3. Visualize that person and imagine that they are in the exact same situation that just caused you to talk so terribly to yourself. Would you say to them what you just said to yourself? Of course you wouldn't.

4. Instead, what would you say to this person, in this circumstance? Inevitably, it would be something kind, loving, and above all, truthful. (Note: be objective and honest here.)

5. Now, say to yourself that exact same thing that you would say to that person. This step may also seem silly to you, but make sure you do it. By telling yourself something true and positive, you are hardwiring those positive feelings about yourself.

6. This takes practice to become a habit. Go through these steps every time you catch yourself saying something mean, negative, or hateful to yourself. The more you do this, the more you will find that instead of speaking badly to yourself, you will get in the habit of saying the things to yourself that you would say to that person you love.

This process is how you will break the bad habit of negative self-talk and over time learn to be your own best friend. Right now you may not be able to imagine the difference eliminating this one bad habit will make, but I promise you it will change the way you feel about yourself and that will pour over into the rest of your life. You will begin to show yourself grace and, more importantly, understand that you deserve to be treated kindly, with love and respect – by yourself as well as by others. You will recall that self-love encompasses thoughts and feelings about yourself. Changing negative self-talk to loving, truthful, positive self-talk is the way you will begin to truly love yourself.

Self-care is how you put self-love into action. Often, we think of things like bubble baths, or walks on the beach, or manicures and pedicures when we think of self-care. And these things are great! It is an amazing thing to take care of your needs and physically nurture yourself. Eating healthy, whole foods is also a practice in self-care. During your eating window, you can eat anything you want. Just because you can do something, doesn't mean you should do it, right? Choosing healthy foods that are delicious and nutritious and make you feel great is an ultimate form of self-care. I used to think making those kinds of choices was "being on a diet." Now I understand that setting healthy boundaries for myself in my food choices demonstrates deep self-love.

What does self-care look like in action? Here are some examples of self-care that underscore your love for yourself.

Self-Care Actions

- Saying positive things to yourself,
- Forgiving yourself when you mess up,
- Knowing what your needs are,
- Meeting your own needs,
- Being assertive and standing up for yourself,
- Not allowing others to take advantage of you,
- Prioritizing your health and well-being,
- Spending time around people who support you and build you up (avoiding those who don't),
- Asking for help,

- Letting go of grudges or anger that hold you back,
- Recognizing and celebrating your strengths,
- Valuing your feelings,
- Making healthy choices a majority of the time,
- Making choices and living according to your own personal values,
- Pursuing your interests and goals,
- Challenging yourself,
- Holding yourself accountable for your actions and choices,
- Giving yourself healthy treats,
- Accepting your imperfections, and loving yourself fully for who you are,
- Setting realistic expectations,
- Noticing your progress and effort and giving yourself credit and acknowledgement for them.

Why do we need self-love to be successful in sustainable weight loss and in reaching our health goals? You can see some of that answer reflected in the list of self-care actions. Without self-love, we are likely to be highly self-critical and fall into people-pleasing perfectionism. We are more likely to make decisions that keep us stuck in obesity and ill health. We may neglect our own needs and feelings because we don't value ourselves. And we may self-sabotage or make decisions that aren't in our own best interest, that don't serve us, and take us farther away from our goals. Self-love is the foundation that allows us to be assertive, set healthy boundaries, practice self-care, pursue our goals, and feel proud of who we are and what we have accomplished.

Chapter 11

MINDSET MATTERS!

A healthy mindset is another one of those elusive puzzle pieces that creates the picture of sustained weight loss and attaining health goals that I was missing all those years. In addition to negative self-talk being a horrible habit, having a negative and destructive mindset is also a terrible, unhealthy bad habit.

Awareness is the first step in turning a bad habit around. I believe awareness comes differently for each of us. In my case, it was when I began to notice how terribly I was speaking to myself. I would get a sick feeling in the pit of my stomach when I noticed it happening; this was my dawning awareness of the problem. Once you become fully aware of an issue, you can choose to turn your bad habits around and develop healthy habits. In fact, the key to making permanent shifts in your mindset is to implement a cycle of improvement.

Here are three simple steps to exchange destructive habits with positive, uplifting habits.

1. Identify what you need to improve – what part of an unhealthy mindset that you want to change,

2. Deliberate practice – focus all your effort on the specific area you want to improve, and

3. Habit – with consistent, intentional practice, the habit will become an automatic action or thought.

During all those years of yo-yo dieting and chasing skinny, I definitely was NOT empowered. *Empowerment – the state of being empowered to do something: the power, right, or authority to do something (*Merriam-Webster dictionary). I did not feel like I had the power to lose weight on my own. I had no feeling of having the authority to make good, healthy choices for myself. Rather, I gave away my power in favor of the endless search for a diet or diet establishment that would take care of me, tell me what to eat and not eat, and how to lose weight. The fact that I chose this action, to give away my power and authority to take care of myself, was a hard but enlightening lesson to learn. For so many years I had a self-deprecating victim mentality. It was the diet establishment's fault that I could never be successful, there was something wrong with all of their diet plans. They were too restrictive, or too hard, or had too many of my favorite foods on the "do not eat" list. It was very sobering to realize that, in fact, I was the problem. However, it was truly empowering when I realized that if I could give away my power, I could certainly take it back.

I am here to share with you the truth. You are not broken. You do not need to be fixed or told what to do. Those were the thoughts and beliefs that I had, and you may be feeling the same thing. You need to take back your power. Just as I discovered about myself, you have the ability, the intelligence, the strength, and the wisdom to make good decisions for yourself about your health and wellness. You are wiser and stronger than you realize. You may not like what you see today, but you can take back your authority, power, and the right to set your own goals, practice intermittent fasting daily, make great food choices most of the time, and enjoy an occasional treat. No one knows you better than you know yourself. You oversee your life, and no-one else can do that for you. Reclaim your power by telling yourself often that you trust yourself to make healthy choices. Listen to what you are telling yourself because, as I always say, "We believe what we tell ourselves."

By telling yourself these things, you are hardwiring in these positive, healthy thoughts and will slowly begin to feel empowered to truly love and care for yourself by taking care of yourself, by making your own decisions about what is best for you. It will take practice, mindfulness, and paying attention to what your body is telling you. The more you practice, the easier it gets.

What foods make you feel alert, energetic, satisfied, and emotionally happy? Which foods cause you to have bloating, headaches, feel shaky or weak, gastric issues, or feeling like you can never be satisfied with what you have eaten? Learning to identify which foods you love and that make you feel great will go a long way in learning to feel that you can trust yourself to make good food and health choices. You do have the power to decide what foods to eat, and what foods work for your body. You'll learn, and the more you practice, you'll find that choosing the right foods for you will become a habit and become ingrained in your daily life. With intermittent fasting, there are no food lists, no good or bad foods. There are foods you enjoy and make you feel great when you eat them. There are tasty treats that you enjoy choosing occasionally. And always, you are in charge and what you eat is your decision. Know that you can and will become empowered to make good choices for you and your body.

Telling myself that I couldn't make good decisions for myself is an example of a self-limiting belief. What are self-limiting beliefs? They are any belief or thought that keeps you from believing that you can be successful in taking charge of your health and life. They are yet another bad habit that we created that has kept us from being successful in sustainable weight loss and in reclaiming our health. They are thoughts and beliefs that come from sad, depressed, negative, defeated feelings. They are not the truth, but we convince ourselves they are. I had so many self-limiting beliefs that I told myself were true. And because we believe what we tell ourselves, I truly did believe these things. Do you share any of these thoughts – do you believe them to be true about yourself?

Self-Limiting Beliefs

- I can't lose weight on my own.
- I'll never be able to lose weight and keep it off.
- I'm a failure; I have failed every weight loss attempt I've ever made.
- I'm going to be fat forever, it's just the way it is.
- It is genetics! I can't control it; how can I control my genes?
- I have no choice; I am going to be overweight forever.
- I might as well eat whatever I want, since I'm always going to be fat anyway.
- It is just not in the cards for me to be a healthy weight.
- No-one will ever love me because I'm fat.
- I might as well quit trying, it never helps.
- If I can't be perfect on my diet, I might as well quit.
- I have to be skinny before I can be in a relationship.
- I can't practice intermittent fasting. I could never go that long without food.
- I could never (fill in the blank) _____ _____.

How many of the 14 bullet points above do you find yourself saying? NONE ARE TRUE.

Part of the responsibility of being empowered to take charge of your life is to be honest with yourself. We all must recognize the fact that all of these are lies that we have told ourselves. They may be what we feel, but they are not the truth. The antidote to self-limiting beliefs is to flip the script and tell ourselves what really is true. Self-honesty is one of those elusive missing puzzle pieces. Telling ourselves the truth is what we have to do to change this bad habit of lying to ourselves, believing things that aren't true that make us feel sad, down, disheartened, and defeated. Truthful thinking is healthy thinking. What does healthy thinking look like? Here are a few examples. Can you think of some more?

- Time is my friend; I know I did not gain this weight overnight, and I know that slow, steady weight loss is the healthiest.
- I make conscious choices about what I am going to eat.
- I own my choices, enjoy whatever I have decided to eat, and move on, feeling content with my choices.
- Some foods serve my body well and make me feel great! Other foods are wonderful to enjoy occasionally for the pure delight of it.
- I eat food for energy, nutrition, to live, to feel well and for life enjoyment. There are no good foods or bad foods.
- I practice intermittent fasting every day. I eat food that I want, food that makes me feel great, and food that I enjoy, all within my daily eating window.
- I DO trust myself to make the best food choices for my body.
- Exercise is a privilege, not a punishment.
- The number on the scale is merely a data point and does not tell the whole story of my health and progress – it is not the best indicator of success.
- Non-scale victories (the way my clothes fit, how I feel, my energy level, my measurements, etc.) are the best and most exciting ways to measure progress.
- _____.
- _____.
- _____.

Continue to practice replacing unhealthy, false, negative thoughts about yourself with healthy thoughts. The more you practice, the sooner healthy thinking will become an automatic habit.

Another type of unhealthy thinking is one I know you will most likely recognize. I often see it referred to as "diet brain" or "diet mentality." I was mired in diet brain for over 40 years. These were thoughts and beliefs that I learned from a young age and they all center around dieting and losing weight. Anyone who shares my history of yo-yo dieting will certainly recognize these disordered thoughts.

➢ I want weight loss results NOW.
➢ If I don't lose lots of weight every week, I am a failure and might as well quit.
➢ I have to be perfect on a diet or I can't be successful.
➢ If I eat "good" food, I am a good person; if I eat "bad" food, I am a bad person.
➢ I have blown it for today and might as well eat whatever I want since I've blown it.
➢ I'll restart my diet next Monday…or next month…or next year.
➢ I have to follow a diet or go to a diet place to lose weight. I can't do it on my own.
➢ Either I am all on my diet or I'm all off.

Collectively, this type of disordered, unhealthy thinking makes up diet brain. It is the kind of thinking that we develop over time with each unsuccessful diet we try. The more diet failures we experience, the more ingrained these types of thoughts become. They did for me, that's for sure. These had been my thoughts for so many years that I didn't even realize they weren't healthy. I didn't realize they weren't true. Diet brain keeps us stuck, doomed to keep repeating the same behaviors while hoping for a different outcome. Diet brain is a specific type of limiting belief.

Once again, the key to eliminating them is to first understand that they are disordered thoughts and not the truth. They are very unhealthy because they affect our behavior and choices, and never for the good. Replacing diet brain thoughts is a matter of recognizing them as they happen, and replacing them with healthy, truthful thoughts. Every time you have one of these untrue thoughts, stop and tell yourself the truth, a healthy thought that is positive, unlike those negative diet brain thoughts. As you see, replacing negative thoughts is an active, intentional practice that takes time and deliberate work. Our thoughts won't change just because we wish they would. It is up to us to become empowered to recognize the problem and do the work to correct it. To change the habit of thinking unhealthy thoughts and replacing them with productive, true, healthy thoughts takes awareness, time, thoughtfulness, commitment, and practice.

The final layer of a healthy mindset is to have a positive attitude. I'm sure you have heard this adage by Henry Ford.

> *"Whether you think you can, or you think you can't, you're right."*
> ~Henry Ford

The truth is, having a positive attitude is a habit. Looking for the positives in a situation didn't come naturally to me. I was much more apt to look at the storm clouds than the silver lining. Looking for the positives in a situation is an intentional act. Thinking positive thoughts is a mindful activity. No one is automatically positive all the time, but we can all cultivate this habit, and become a person who's automatically positive most of the time. Habit Regulation, the process of intentionally developing habits by using repetition, is in part dependent on feelings of positivity. Who could eliminate an unhealthy habit or begin good habits if they weren't feeling positive and optimistic about their ability to make those shifts happen?

Nobody disputes that a positive mindset is a crucial shift to achieving long-term health and weight loss goals. I can guarantee you that each time I "fell off the diet wagon" and sank into the familiar downward spiral of unhealthy choices and weight regain – my thoughts were incredibly negative. Bad days happen too, right? Who can be positive all the time? I sure wasn't. We can all recognize that not every day is a great day, but if we are intentional and decide to do it, we can all find some good in every day, even when you have to look pretty hard to find it. To cultivate a positive attitude is not to bury your head in the sand, however. Recognizing that a day isn't a good day is truthful, but if you decide to look for positive things, you can always find something, even on difficult days. And doing so gives you a boost like you wouldn't believe. Intentional positivity truly makes a difference in our mood and how we feel. And if yesterday wasn't such a great day and you found it difficult to find a single positive thing about it? Decide not to let a bad day yesterday ruin a good day today by dwelling on it. Let it go! The more you practice being positive with intention, the more automatic these thoughts will become.

A positive attitude is extremely helpful when making food choices in your window. I got into the habit of asking myself, "Does this choice support my goals? Will it get me closer to reaching my goal or move me further away from reaching it?" Our weight loss goals support our overarching goals of enjoying great health, overall wellness, and a feeling of contentment with our bodies and our lives.

I found that a positive attitude helped me with one of the most challenging aspects of weight loss, being patient. I needed to understand that I didn't become obese and unhealthy overnight, and that I had to accept that reversing these conditions was going to take time and patience. We won't reach our weight loss goals overnight, but if we give up, it won't happen at all. Positive thinking gave me the ability to appreciate that a little progress each day added up to big results. While the magic of intermittent fasting is in the clean fast, patience was the 'secret sauce' that allowed the magic to happen for me, over time.

Additionally, having a positive attitude was key in realizing that my non-scale victories (NSVs) were critical in my motivation and day-to-day happiness. They were truly the good stuff in my weight loss journey, and by noticing and celebrating these accomplishments, small and large, I nourished myself and became able to practice that patience, which I previously always found to be practically impossible.

Don't be discouraged by the work that is involved in changing habits. Take your time, be consistent and intentional in your work, and celebrate every time you think positive, healthy thoughts and make healthy choices. Make sure to forgive yourself and give yourself grace when you miss the mark, because we all miss the mark at times. Over time these good habits will become automatic. And these are the changes that we all must make to have sustainable weight loss and in finding great health long term. Along with practicing intermittent fasting as a permanent lifestyle, of course!

It's time to become your own best friend.

Chapter 12

MOVEMENT: THE OTHER FOUNTAIN OF YOUTH

I hated gym class when I was in school. Always did. I wasn't overweight as a child, but I was very shy. I was always the last picked for teams. It was embarrassing and hurt my feelings deeply. I was also very uncoordinated and hated getting all sweaty, plus I was a reader, not an active kid, so I could never keep up when we played strenuous games. This trend continued as I got older. I really didn't ever get into sports, and exercise for health certainly wasn't on my radar. The closest I came to ever liking any kind of physical activity was swimming and diving, which I actually excelled at every summer (too bad we didn't have swimming or diving classes in school!), and hiking with my Girl Scout® troop. These activities were fun. I loved being out in the woods, I loved when the troop leaders would point out all kinds of interesting wildlife while we were hiking and, of course, the campfire featuring S'mores later in the evening. I also loved that I felt a part of the gang and was included. It didn't take any kind of strength or coordination to walk on the trails, and without realizing it, I was getting in all kinds of great movement on our hikes.

Fast-forward to adulthood. I worked, put myself through college, and got married. I had started gaining weight by this point, and the great hunt for the perfect diet was well underway. It was at this time that I also started trying to lose weight by joining gyms. Although now that I think about it, the first fad exercise solution I tried to lose weight was with my mom during my high school years, because she asked me

Chapter 12 | Movement: the Other Fountain of Youth

to. I can't remember the name of the gym, but it was for women only and everything inside of it was pink. Pink carpet, pink walls, pink exercise equipment. I guess if you didn't like pink, you were out of luck.

You got on a machine, and they put this belt around your hips, and it vibrated. We called it the fat jiggler machine. It was expensive, embarrassing, and ineffective. That was the end of my trying to exercise until I began to really gain weight. As I was trying different diets, I joined various gyms. I would go for a while. The truth is, down deep I really didn't want to go. But I did want to lose weight, so I would start out gung-ho, all in, doing way too much too fast. It wouldn't take me long to hurt myself or get completely worn out and start skipping exercise classes or sessions, and that would be the end of that gym. I bought exercise equipment for home like jump ropes and expensive running shoes. For a while I remember jogging around the block and working my way up to several times around. But my interest in that quickly faded because I just didn't like doing it. It was a chore, and I didn't like chores, so I quit. For more years than I care to remember, I was joining diet programs and gyms and quitting each one within a few months. It became part of that sad diet cycle that I never seemed to be able to escape. I always focused on cardio and never attempted any kind of weight training. I saw no need for that.

Fast-forward again, and you will find me well into losing weight through my intermittent fasting practice. At 56 and well past menopause, I had healed several health conditions, lost almost 55 pounds within 6 months (I went on to lose a total of 110 pounds over 14 months), and lo and behold I was feeling the old familiar pull to exercise. I finally wanted to exercise, but what to do? I didn't care to join a gym. Looking back, I realize that the problem that I had been having with self-limiting beliefs had spilled over into my thinking pertaining to exercise. I had several self-limiting beliefs that had always held me back in the area of exercise.

I am thinking that since I suffered from these self-limiting beliefs, you may share some of these same thoughts about exercise right now.

- If you aren't sweating, you aren't doing any good.
- Exercise is punishment for eating bad food.
- Exercise is a total chore.
- Exercise is boring.
- Exercise is too hard!
- If I eat too much of something I shouldn't, I have to work it off with lots of extra exercise.
- Exercise is only for young people or athletes.
- I have to join a gym to exercise and it's too expensive.
- Exercise takes too long – it has to be done in a big chunk of time.
- I don't have time to exercise.

In Chapter 11, I shared that self-limiting beliefs are false statements. I want you to read back through these self-limiting beliefs regarding exercise and turn them around. Choose 7 that you currently tell yourself and write them under SELF-LIMITING BELIEF in the chart below. Then write the truth beside each one; it will be the opposite of what is written.

SELF-LIMITING BELIEF	TRUTH/OPPOSITE
1.	1.
2.	2.
3.	3.
4.	4.
5.	5.
6.	6.
7.	7.

If you are like me, even the word "exercise" evokes negative emotions, like those bad memories of gym class in school or being forced to play games and participate in sports that I didn't enjoy. Within that sentence is a big part of the problem… "being forced to play games and sports that I didn't enjoy." When we were in school, we had no choice or ability to decide what activities would most suit us. I hated being forced to play games that I wasn't successful at, and it set me up for a lifetime of hating sports.

Likely after school and over the weekend you were out playing with your friends, doing things you loved, and no-one had to make you do it. You just did what was fun and did not think about it being "exercise." So, let's ditch that word exercise and think instead about fun, healthy movement. Some people love to go hard, work up a sweat, feel the burn, and continually beat their own personal bests. For them, that is the true essence of fun movement. It is what they love to do, and that is great! For another person, this same regimen might be torture. A walk while listening to energetic music or a podcast is a great movement plan for this person. After all, the best exercise is the exercise you will actually do.

First, let's talk cardio. Finding a way to integrate enjoyable movement into your day is important for your overall health and wellness. It promotes stress reduction, mental clarity, heart health, and helping prevent future disease. What fulfilling movement means to you is personal and will be different for each of us. I shared my story earlier about walking, listening to my beloved playlist, and becoming a fitness walker. I love that! It is something that I look forward to and I especially love how it makes me feel. It reminds me of the hiking I did as a Girl Scout®.

Many people say they hate exercise (myself included). But when asked to think of what they loved to do as a child or what kind of play they engaged in with their friends, adults often animatedly speak of their great childhood and all of the fun they had. Bike riding often comes up, as does swimming, running, climbing trees, playing informal sports games with the neighborhood gang, and hiking. Many have fond memories of various movement activities; they just don't think of them as exercise. How about you? What kinds of things did you love to do, either in gym class or after school and on the weekends with your friends or family?

It's time to play again. Thinking back on your childhood will help point you in the right direction. Were you more of a team-oriented kid, or did you enjoy solo activities? Be open to new ideas! Try a kickboxing class, yoga, tai chi, swimming laps, water aerobics, or chair yoga. Maybe playing 18 holes gets your juices flowing. Or are you more practically minded? Do you love doing some serious cleaning, including washing walls and hosing down patios? Does gardening, mowing, trimming, and raking leaves in your yard fit the bill? Or do you love to run and play with your grandchildren? The point is, any of these things count as healthy movement, especially when they are things you love to do. Just keep looking until you find movement to incorporate into your life that invigorates and energizes you, something you look forward to. Ultimately, you are in charge of your own health, and finding movement you enjoy is your responsibility. So have fun as you solve this puzzle for yourself. Continue to cultivate a positive mindset and approach your search with a sense of wonder and excitement. If you try something and do not enjoy it, no big deal. Keep experimenting! The only way you can fail is if you just give up. While cardio is important for heart and lung efficiency, it is strength training that provides the benefits that keep our body younger, stronger, and more functional as each year passes by. If we want to be vibrant and independent for many more years, strength training will help us achieve just that.

Strength training is important for everyone, especially for women after 50 as it becomes even more crucial than ever. It isn't about having big biceps or flat abs, but rather takes on a tone of maintaining a strong, healthy body that is less prone to injury and illness. Strength training after 50 helps our body in the following ways:

*Builds Bone Density

Unexpected falls put countless older people in the hospital every year. An 8-year-old boy gets a cast on his arm and gets back to playing in 8 weeks. A 70-year-old isn't quite so fortunate. The ramifications of broken bones can be horrible. Strength training can help.

*Builds Muscle Mass

No, this does not mean you will turn into the Incredible Hulk. It means that you will be a solid, strong person who can lift their own groceries, push their own lawnmower, and pick yourself up if you fall. Living independently as long as we can is the goal.

*Decreases Body Fat

Too much body fat isn't ideal for any of us, at any age. Maintaining a healthy weight, in conjunction with living your intermittent fasting lifestyle, is important especially when it comes to preventing many diseases that come with aging populations.

*Improves Mental Health

Along with aging comes a higher rate of depression and, for many, a loss of self-confidence. Strength training has been shown to improve your general sense of accomplishment and can help you experience improved confidence and well-being.

*Lowers the Risk of Chronic Disease

The Centers for Disease Control and Prevention® (CDC®) recommends strength training for most older adults to help lessen the symptoms of the following chronic conditions: arthritis, osteoporosis, diabetes, obesity, back pain, and depression.

*Must-Do Strength Training Moves for Women Over 50, VeryWellFit.com, 2021.

Strength training is a pretty good deal. For just 20-30 minutes a day, you can see big changes in your body's age. And you don't need to, nor should you, use heavy weights. Use very light weights and few repetitions. I started with one-pound dumbbells just to get me started. I very slowly increased my weight and reps, and I have never done very heavy weights. You do you. There are dumbbells, medicine balls, kettlebells, stretch bands, and other types of strength training equipment. Do your research and, most importantly, start very slowly. Before starting any diet or exercise routine, check with your doctor.

With intermittent fasting and strength training both described as the fountain of youth, what are you waiting for?

EPILOGUE

*"You must be big enough to admit your mistakes, smart
enough to learn from them, and strong enough
to correct them."*
~John C. Maxwell

The past few years have been filled with exponential growth in my life. I learned I had strength that I never knew I had. I learned that I could be empowered to take charge of my life instead of letting food control me. I learned that my mindset was my biggest problem and had led to health issues that I never dreamed I would have at such a young age, and that menopause does not mean the end of the road. I discovered an amazing lifestyle, intermittent fasting, that when lived with consistency, brings true holistic healing and a beautiful sense of food freedom, peacefulness, and contentment to our lives, regardless of what weight you do or do not need to lose.

I also learned that no matter how high you climb, it is possible to have a fall. That life nor weight loss are straight lines; life happens, and we don't always deal with it in the manner that we wish we would have. The last year was like that for me. I really stumbled and took a wild ride on the struggle bus! I would not publish this book without being 100% honest and transparent. Pure and simple, I started doing some things and stopped doing some things and gained some weight back. I don't deal with the scale much, it took me a very long time to break free of the scales' hold on me, but my clothes told the tale of what I already knew. I started making bad choices, and I'm afraid I did that rather consistently for quite a while.

I am all about taking responsibility for my choices and actions. This epilogue is not meant to be a boo-hoo, poor me pity party. It is meant to show that we all can make mistakes, take a step in the wrong direction, and still be okay. It is to demonstrate that while things may not always be perfect, that we are perfectly capable of turning it around by using the tools in our intermittent fasting toolkit, our experience with success, and by simply making the decision to get back to what we know works – truly living an intermittent fasting lifestyle with consistency. After all, consistency is the one thing that can overcome any obstacle.

This quote by John C. Maxwell has been my blueprint for turning it around, and it is my blueprint for writing this epilogue.

My Mistakes

My very first mistake was to let stress affect my choices, and I returned to the bad habit of emotional eating. A year-long, difficult job as a COVID-19 screener and supervisor at a hospital, way too much overtime, and a sad personal situation all led to months of tremendous stress. I eventually got back into the bad habit of eating for comfort, not nutrition. Author James Clear is so right when he says that habits drive our lives. I saw it happening but was in denial and thought I could turn it around anytime, but once we allow bad habits to control us, we have totally lost control.

My other mistake was to let emotion get involved, which exacerbated the bad habits that I had slipped back into, such as too much sugar, unhealthy and unwise food choices way too often, and having very short fasts consistently. I never quit intermittent fasting, but I certainly didn't practice it faithfully, for many months. Bad habits led to panic over the choices I was making and the weight I was gaining, which led to more bad eating habits. I got mostly into the bad habit of making unhealthy choices based on emotion. On top of all of that, I gradually quit exercising, which had done so many great things for my physical and emotional health.

Lessons Learned and Corrective Actions

Probably one of the hardest things to face during this time was that I had stopped being honest with myself. Learning to tell myself what is true, not lies based on negative emotion, was a very hard-won lesson for me to learn as I lost weight and gained knowledge and perspective. That was the first thing I changed; my first lesson learned. Do NOT allow yourself to be in denial. I had to tell myself the truth, and admit that I was choosing these actions, they weren't something that just 'happened to me' because I went through a rough patch.

Next, I had to reidentify the bad habits that I picked back up during this difficult time and reverse them. I had to go through the process of eliminating bad eating habits and creating my healthy habits again. The good news is that I knew how to do it, I just had to make the decision to do it. It wasn't always easy, but we know that habit change can be one of the hardest things that we need to do to live an intermittent fasting lifestyle.

Another lesson learned was to get back to my 20/4 protocol, every day. And it came back fairly easily, to my delight. I really did deeply ingrain some fantastic habits as I lost weight, and although I spent some time away from them, they came back easily. Getting rid of the bad habits, however, was much harder. I learned to be vigilant about my habits, both good and bad, because they determine my success! Another thing I did to help myself was to get a fantastic accountability partner. She is supportive while still asking the hard questions, and we have been great for each other. Together we are going to reach the goals we have set for ourselves.

And finally, I am waiting for the go-ahead from my orthopedic surgeon to get back to walking, after a recent hip-replacement surgery. The next thing I will be adding back is light resistance training, and that is coming soon!

Mostly, I want you to know that it is possible that you, too, may go through some difficult times. You probably won't always be perfect, you could gain a few pounds, or more, back. Or you might not! What I most want you to know is that you ALWAYS have intermittent fasting. It will never fail you, and you do have the strength, knowledge, and the experience to make a course correction if it is ever needed. Because, after all, the only way you can fail is if you quit. And I know that just like me, you will never be a quitter!

As a certified health and life coach, specializing in intermittent fasting and mindset work, my virtual coaching business provides coaching services to those who want to finally lose weight and become healthy and happy. This book closely follows along with my 12-week coaching program. If you're ready to change your life forever, go to my website, www.fastingwithpaige.com, and let's get started. I'm here to help you every step of the way.

Paige

www.ingramcontent.com/pod-product-compliance
Lightning Source LLC
Chambersburg PA
CBHW020300030426
42336CB00010B/838